Dancing Your Way to Fertility Bonus Book: How I Had the Babies of My Dreams and How You Can Too—Plus The Ultimate Fertility Success Program!

Dancing Your Way to Fertility
Paula Fuoco Davis
PaulaMediaandEntertainment.com, Nashua, NH
Edition Notice 1
Date of Publication Nov. 10, 2016
Number of Printings: First printing
Year of publication: 2016

This book is not intended to be a substitute for the medical advice of a licensed physician. The reader should consult with their doctor in any matters relating to his/her health.

The author and publisher expressly disclaim responsibility for any adverse effect that may result from the use or application of the information contained in this book.

As an express condition to reading this book, and associated products, you must agree to the following terms. If you disagree with any of these terms, please do not read this book. Your use of this book, its website or products means that you are agreeing to be legally bound by these terms.

You agree to hold this book, LLC, its owners, agents, and employees harmless from any and all liability for all claims for damages due to injuries, including attorney fees and costs, incurred by you or caused to third parties by you, arising out of the information discussed in this book.

We make no representation or warranties with respect to the accuracy or completeness of the contents of this book and we specifically disclaim any implied warranties of merchantability.

This book does not contain all information available on this subject. This book has not been created to be specific to any individual's or organizations' situation or needs. This book should not be considered as the ultimate source of subject information. This book contains information that might be dated.

All material in this book is provided as information only and may not be construed as medical advice or instruction. No action or inaction should be taken based solely on the contents of this book. Instead, readers should consult appropriate health professionals on any matter relating to their health and well-being.

Reliance on any information provided by the author and this book is solely at your own risk.

The material in this book is provided for informational purposes only and is not intended as medical advice. The information contained in this book should not be used to diagnose or treat any illness, disorder, disease or health problem. Use of the programs, advice, and information contained in this book is at the sole choice and risk of the reader.

The resources and information made available in this book are provided for informational purposes only, and should not be used to replace the specialized training and professional judgment of a health care or mental health care professional.

The author and publisher cannot be held responsible for the use of the information provided. Please always consult a physician or a trained mental health professional before making any decision regarding treatment of yourself or others.

If you are currently in treatment or in therapy, please consult your therapist, psychiatrist or mental health professional before you use any of the information contained in this book.

If you feel suicidal or depressed, contact a Crisis Hotline or seek help at a hospital, Emergency Room, treatment center, or with a physician, qualified mental health care provider, or through a law enforcement agency or social services.

This book and its contents (including any information available from the book located on websites or excerpted) is for informational and entertainment purposes only and is not intended to replace or substitute for any professional, medical, legal, mental health or any other advice.

In addition, the author and publisher make no representations or warranties and expressly disclaims any and all liability concerning any treatment or action by any person following the information offered or provided within or through this book. If you have specific concerns or find yourself in a situation in which you require professional or medical advice, you should consult with an appropriately trained and qualified specialist.

Please consult your physician, mental health professional or therapist before you utilize the materials that can be purchased from this book.

If you do not agree to be bound by all of these terms, do not read this book.

We make no representation or warranties with respect to the accuracy or completeness of the contents of the book and we specifically disclaim any implied warranties of merchantability for any particular purpose.

All material in this book is provided for your information only and may not be construed as medical advice or instruction. No action or inaction should be taken based on the contents of this information. Instead, readers should consult appropriate health professionals on any matter relating to their health and well-being.

The information in this book does not and is not intended to replace professional medical or nutritional advice.

The information contained in this book should not be considered complete and does not cover all diseases, ailments, physical conditions or their treatment. It should not be used in place of a call or visit to a medical,health or other competent professional, who should be consulted beforeadopting any of the suggestions in this book or drawing inferences from it.

The information about drugs, herbs, vitamins, foods, drinks, and any other food sources contained in this book is general in nature.

They do not cover all possible uses, actions, precautions, side effects, or interactions of the medicines mentioned, nor is the information intended as medical advice for individual problems or for making an evaluation as to the risks and benefits of taking a particular drug, vitamin, herb, supplement, or food.

This book and the operator(s) of this site specifically disclaim all responsibility for any liability, loss or risk, personal or otherwise, which is incurred as a consequence, directly or indirectly, of the use and application of any of the material on this site.

If you do anything recommended in this book without the supervision of a licensed medical doctor, you do so at your own risk because the information, remedies or exercise in this book may not be U.S. Food and Drug Administration (FDA) approved.

The medical information in this book is provided "as is" without any representations or warranties, express or implied.

You must not rely on the information in this book as an alternative to medical advice from your doctor or other professional health care provider.

If you think you may be suffering from any medical condition or before starting any new treatment you should seek immediate medical attention. Proper medical attention should always be sought for specific ailments.

Never disregard professional medical advice, delay in seeking medical treatment or discontinue medical treatment due to information obtained in this book

Any information provided in this book is not intended to diagnose, treat or cure infertility or any other illness, disease or medical condition.

Books may be purchased by contacting the publisher and author at books@paulamediaandentertainment.com.

Books may be purchased in quantity and/or special sales by contacting the publisher, PaulaMediaandEntertainment.com or by email at books@paulamediaandentertainment.com.

Library of Congress Catalog Number:
ISBN:
1. Infertility 2. Fertility 3. Health

First Edition

This book is dedicated to my mother, Sarah Fuoco for being the best mother in the world. You embody what motherhood is in every way. I have always loved and will always love sitting across from you at the kitchen table talking. There is no place I rather be. I loved as a child seeing your white car waiting to pick me up from school, our Monday trips to the mall, visits to Friendlys, and every moment inbetween. You were kind when I didn't deserve it, and more loving and amazing then I could have ever hoped for. I am grateful you are my Mom. How could I not want to be a mother after having a mother like you? You gave me everything and more and I can't thank you enough for being everything to me.

My father, Joseph Fuoco, for taking such good care of me and Mom, and working so hard and responsibly to make life beautiful for us. You were a fun Dad, smart, generous and loving. How can I even begin to thank you for all you have given me? Thank you for paying for all my vitamins as I went through infertility treatments. For this, I could never say thank you enough. You are a beautiful person.

My beautiful children, Amber and Sammy, who God sent as an answer to all my prayers. You were worth every part of this journey, every needle, every minute..all so worth it because having you both has been the most wonderful part of my life. You both fill my days with more joy than you can imagine. Amber, from the day you were born, I saw you as gold from heaven. You are the perfect girl for me. I like and love everything about you. Thank you for all the conversations—you are never boring and I needed that in my life so much. Thank you for loving books and being such a great writer that you constantly surprise me with your ability—and thank you for sitting on my lap for hours as a baby and toddler and letting me read to you. Those moments were pure joy. Sammy, (whose friends also know as Brandon) from the moment you were born, you were glistening with a perfect sweetness. You were the boy I needed in my life always. Thanks for playing baseball with me. You, like your sister, are like gold to me. You are understanding, smart, handsome and fun—who would have ever imagined I would have a son so good at basketball? Amber and Sammy, thank you for everything….all the great car rides to Grandma's where you put up with my changing the radio station every five minutes and everything else. You are both amazing, beautiful, and so smart. I am beyond privileged to be your mother.

Most of all, I dedicate this book to Jehovah God, the one who answers all prayers. Thank you, thank you, thank you Jehovah. Without you, I could not have survived this. Without the privilege of prayer, I would not have been able to walk this road. Without you, all this would have never happened. Thank you for listening, for always being there, and for helping me have the babies of my dreams. I could never thank you enough. There is no God like you, and you deserve every bit of praise and honor always.

My best friend, Leah Page Mortimer, who walked with me and helped me every step of the way. You were there during my darkest times, offering hope, acceptance, love, understanding. Yes, you are a genius! And for all the times you said exactly what I needed to hear, thank you.

My husband, Christopher Davis, for being there and walking this hard road with me. You were brave and kind, a true hero, and without you, I would not have my kids. There is no one else I would have rather walked this road with. You helped me give birth to these beautiful children and I can't thank you enough.

Table of Contents

I suffered and cried, but in the end my dream came true.

I want the same to happen to you.

I tried to put in this book everything I wish someone told me, so my journey would not have been so painful, and maybe I would have been successful a little bit sooner.

I wish you all the success you deserve.

Paula Fuoco Davis: For more than 30 years, she worked as a newspaper reporter and journalist for The Lawrence Eagle-Tribune, The Nashua Telegraph and New Hampshire magazine. She covered education, social issues and features. She founded and is editor of Commitment.com, an online site for women and authored more than 25 books. She is a survivor of infertility and wants others to have every single bit of information she didn't have. She has loved writing this book.

Dancing Your Way to Fertility Bonus Book: A condensed version of the original to enjoy.

If you want to read the entire version, Dancing Your Way to Fertility can be purchased at Amazon.com or at www.dancingyourwaytofertility.com.

Dancing Your Way to Fertility

My doctor looked at me point blank and said without a trace of mercy that my eggs were "bottom of the barrel."

Bottom of the barrel... Her words rang in my head like a cruel pronouncement.

I was 37 years old and desperately wanted a second child. My doctor didn't believe I could have one.

I had been through this before. To have my daughter, I endured 10 IUIs, several operations and too many nights of crying to count.

So I left her office: desperate, heartbroken, and wildly, frantically panicked. The words 'your eggs are bottom of the barrel' kept repeating in my head. Despite everything I've gone through, I always had hope. My insides were screaming: 'I can't live with this.' I was so shaken, I could barely drive home. Her words nearly broke my will and spirit to try again.

For some reason, on the way home, I stopped at a natural foods market. Walking around the supermarket, amidst all the healthy foods and supplements, I began to question what the doctor told me. Was the poor quality of my eggs something that could be improved? Was I unhealthy on some undetectable level that was impacting my fertility? I went home and called my ever-wise mother. She gave me great advice: dump that doctor and try again.

I did exactly what Mom said.

I decided I would do everything I could to restore and heal my fertility, and not be hindered by my age, regardless of what the doctor said.

Over time, I learned that there was hope for me and others like me—and just because a doctor says you can never get pregnant does not mean your body, if given the right elements, cannot heal from infertility.

My devastation and despair turned to determination, and everything I learned, I put in this book. As a newspaper reporter for more than 25 years, I utilized my skills as a journalist to get to the root of fertility problems, the physical and the emotional.

I am now also a fertility success certified life coach.

I wrote this book for those of you suffering with infertility, who like me who have been told that your eggs are too old, that your body is too unhealthy, weak, or damaged, that there is little hope.

I wrote this book for all of you who feel that having a child is some type of impossible dream, that you are the victim of some pathologically cruel biological problem.

I wrote it for you brave survivors of infertility who dream of starting a family, but find the road long, cruel, uphill, and not always forgiving of slight mistakes and accumulated years.

Together, we will work to heal everything in your body and mind that could be stopping you from getting pregnant. Consider me your personal fertility success coach.

I will help you identify all the physical and emotional obstacles that might be standing in the way of your having the children you desire. Then-one-by-one, we are going to knock these obstacles out of your body and your life.

I created the Ultimate Fertility Success Program, which I believe is one of the most comprehensive body-mind makeover plans available to fertility patients today.

The Ultimate Fertility Success Program includes 12 cleanses that will detoxify your body and expand your fertility potential.

It will also show you how to improve the quality of your eggs—something previously not thought possible—and balance your hormones.

It includes a chapter on strengthening, preparing, and emotionally and spiritually healing every organ in your body that impacts your fertility.

Then we will look at the foods you eat, the lifestyle you live, and vitamins and herbs that will give you a fair and fighting chance to enjoy vibrant fertility. You may be eating, thinking and experiencing life in a way that is depleting your reproductive organs, and you didn't even know it.

The program is designed to change the track you are on so you can become more healthy, vibrant and fertile—as you deserve to be!

For your guy, I've included The Ultimate Male Fertility Preparation Plan, that includes little known information to help your guy enhance his fertility.

We will address all the obvious and not so obvious blocks to your fertility, because some fertility problems are difficult to diagnose and there are not yet diagnostic tools available to detect the slight shifts, blocks, and traumas in the body that can prevent or delay pregnancy.

The traumas and painful emotions we experience can lodge themselves in our cells, interrupting our body's natural healthy energy flow.

This book will help you examine all aspects of your life, from your childhood and family experiences, to your deepest thoughts and beliefs about pregnancy and motherhood, so that you are fully aware of your subconscious feelings and beliefs and every part of you can work together to have the babies of your dreams.

I will share with you the information you need to unblock and destroy the emotional and spiritual traumas, thoughts and fears that could secretly be preventing your body from having a baby.

I've included 50 art, writing, music and dance activities you can do in your home to help you unlock your creative reproductive powers and release negative energy patterns in your body.

Everything in this book can be used in conjunction with an IVF, IUI or other assisted reproductive technologies. We will discuss how to prepare for an IUI and/or IVF, and how to treat yourself the days following these procedures to maximize your chances of getting pregnant.

I have included my own story of battling infertility that I hope you will find useful and inspiring.

As a bonus, I'm including:

• Your Fertility Food Tracker Diary: Its simple, easy to use and will help you track what fertility foods you are giving your body each day.

I've also included several other free journals. These include:

• Journal Writing Through Your Subconscious: to help you discover what your deepest consciousness truly thinks about fertility, motherhood and parenting.

• Your Daily Happiness Journal: to help you gain access to your inner positive-feeling antenna that is ever alert to everything good within you and around you.

• Life Affirmation Journal: designed to help you take note of all the ways birth and life take place in the world around you each day, and how you are intrinsically part of the world's never-ending reproductive cycle.

• My Child & I Journal: where you can share your dreams of a future with your children by your side.

• Emotional Tracking Journal: to help you understand what triggers your positive and negative emotions each day.

This book will also discuss how to:

• Deal with negative comments from friends and relatives, as well as your own internal negativity.

• How to not let infertility ruin your marriage.

• How to choose the right doctor and clinic.

• Ways to reduce stress in your life.

• Writing exercises that will give you a chance to go deep within to unearth and destroy all the self-defeating beliefs and traumas that might be buried deep in your tissues that could be destroying your fertility.

• More than 100 affirmations and visualizations.

• A personal fertility vision statement, that I have written as a certified life coach. It is used to help motivate and get you past the blocks and obstacles to your fertility. You can listen to and read it each day.

• Letters you can send yourself, or just leave around the house, when you need a lift or a reminder of how strong and powerful you really are.

• How to start enjoying a close loving friendship with your body, so your body becomes your best friend and teammate.

• How to turn your home into a fertility nesting center.

• Coping with the unfairness of it all.

- **Ways to protect your baby once you are pregnant**

And all my mistakes (which were many) you can learn from.

This is, most importantly, a book of hope...and about taking action to have the children you deserve and are worthy of.

That doctor who claimed my eggs were 'bottom of the barrel' was wrong. Less than a year later, I gave birth to my beautiful son.

Someday, I would like to send her a picture of my boy and write in blazing letters across the picture: "Is this what bottom of the barrel looks like?"

Infertility: A Training Ground for Motherhood?

 In times past, women have always endured sacrifice and trial as part of motherhood. Now, due to a host of factors such as age, health and environment, women are put through a severe test of their maternal stamina even before they conceive their child.

This road, this test, this initiation, will test all of you--and it will make you one of the strongest, most capable, confident, resourceful, perseverant mothers a child could ever have. Experiencing infertility gives you a lifetime pass to enjoy motherhood in a way few ever get to enjoy it, because with the difficulties of this disease come confidence and appreciation.

 This journey will demand all the best parts of you. It will demand you persevere when you want to give up. It will demand patience and persistence when frustration and helpless surrender might feel like a more natural path. It will demand that every survival skill you possess be brought forth and utilized. It will demand sacrifice, self-preservation, and a willpower beyond what you knew you had, but what intrinsically you knew you were capable of.

If you are not fortunate, you may have your heart broken in 1000 pieces.

If you are fortunate, you could still have your heart broken in 1000 places.

When you give birth to your baby none of it will matter. Your heart will heal, the scars will seem insignificant, and all the tears, disappointments and devastations will seem like bunny rabbits and balloons on a summer's day.

No big deal.

If you do not give birth to a baby, but decide to adopt, become a foster parent, a teacher, coach, counselor or play a very active role in the life of a young niece, nephew, neighbor, or cousin, you will be ready and able to mother these children and impact a younger generation in a way more powerful than you ever imagined.

You have probably been through the best training course for motherhood possible: you understand pain, you understand the potential for joy, you are willing to do the work to get the child you want, and you've proven you can take the bad stuff that comes with going after the good stuff. In doing this, you will join a group of super cultivated mothers, women ready to nurture and love the next generation, and have more than proven their worth to do this.

Infertility hurts.

Winning over infertility can be a painful process that demands resolve and sacrifice.

It is an initiation rite, of sorts, an involuntary one, of course. No one should have to go through this to have a baby and no one would voluntarily choose this road. Nonetheless, it is a reality for many of us, and it will prepare you for motherhood in a grand and inspiring way that someday you may even feel thankful to have experienced.

It is a long road and an unfair one, but at the end of the road, you could be holding the baby of your dreams, just as the same as someone who made love one night and woke up pregnant the next morning.

Then nothing at all will matter but your baby.

Ten Things About Infertility That Nobody Will Tell You-- But You Need To Know Right From The Start

1. You are going to hear no. Expect to hear it at times, but don't let hearing it keep you down or stop you from going after your dream.

2. You are going to have to put some aspects of your life on hold. It will be worth it, but be prepared to spend your time, energy and money on getting pregnant and putting certain aspects of your life on hold.

3. You are going to hear negative comments, sometimes even from the people you love. Don't pay attention to what they say. This can work out for you, despite what anyone says or thinks about your health or situation.

4. This is a journey you might sometimes take alone. Don't be surprised if sometimes even your husband can't be there for you the way you need him to. If that happens, don't waste your time getting angry--just keep going.

5. The doctor you choose and the reproductive clinic they are associated with matters—choose a good one. You want a doctor who is open to trying new medications and procedures and who answers your questions and listens to what you have to say.

6. You are going to have to eat and take care of your body in a way you never have before. Get ready to make spinach, garlic and pumpkin seeds your new best friends.

7. You are going to have to be strong and stay positive, even when nothing positive is happening. You are going to have to get ready to harness every little bit of inner strength you've ever had.

8. You are also going to fall apart sometimes. Just expect it.

9. It is going to feel rotten to be invited to baby showers, children's parties, and see pregnant women at the supermarket. When that happens, just remember: someday, it could very well be you having that baby shower, hosting the children's parties and being that beautiful pregnant lady at the supermarket. And you never know: that mother with the beautiful baby that made your heart ache? She might have once been a fertility patient too.

10. You are going to have to work hard and be flexible. It is important to understand that a lot of work may be required to beat infertility. Infertility treatments require going to lots of appointments, and doing whatever you can to improve your health. This journey takes effort and push. Accepting the hard work involved will make it easier, and hopefully empower you to do what is available to heal your infertility. While beating infertility can be really hard work, the reward it well worth any effort you have to make.

Chapter 1: The Ultimate Fertility Success Program: Getting Your Body Ready

Are you ready to be pregnant? Have you been told that you cannot get pregnant for unexplainable reasons? Have you been trying for a baby for a long time and you are weary, tired and very, very sad?

Infertility is one of the most difficult journeys a woman can take.

But, starting today, know this: Infertility is not a final statement on your ability to have the family you dream of—infertility is a medical condition that, with the right treatments, is often temporary and can be cured.

So starting today, see your infertility as a temporary condition that is a signal that your body is off-track and needs something to heal it.

Infertility clinics often give patents a diagnosis of "unexplained infertility", but infertility is never a result of unexplainable, mysterious problems. Infertility is always a result of specific problems or deficits in the body—problems that are sometimes hard to detect in the way that Western medicine diagnoses ailments.

When your body does not conceive easily and naturally, there is disease, dysfunction and malfunction occurring on some level, even if it is a level so very subtle that it cannot be detected on standardized tests.

Some of the fertility problems your body may be experiencing may be hard to find because there are not machines or diagnostic tools yet available to detect slight shifts, blocks, traumas in the body that can prevent or delay pregnancy.

So just because a doctor says you can never get pregnant does not mean your body, if helped, cannot heal from infertility—but here's the catch—you have to do the right things to get back your infertility.

By turning your body from acidic to alkaline, from a diseased toxic state to one that is cleansed, from a body full of inflammation to one that is healthy.

Sometimes, our body can get onto a disease track, and it then must be pushed and healed back over to a track of health.

In this chapter, we'll discuss a comprehensive body makeover program that will change the track you are on and help you become more healthy, vibrant and fertile—as you deserve to be!

You can go to an infertility clinic and take advantage of all the latest and best treatments and medications available, which I recommend, and at the same time embark on a course of holistic, alternative healing to maximize your chances of getting pregnant and having the babies you dream of.

The first step to overcoming infertility is to change the track your body is on from:

• A state of disease and dysfunction to one of health

• An acidic state to an alkaline state

• A state of clogged toxins in the body, to one of a cleansed body with all your organs cleansed and able to function at their highest level possible.

What can set the body down a wrong course? Unhealthy foods, low-quality drinking water, chemicals or toxins in our environment and in products we use, stress, traumas and painful life experiences that tire and weaken our organs.

Sometimes we live, eat, think and experience life in a way that can deplete our reproductive organs in ways that we are completely unaware of.

Picture yourself driving down the highway in the wrong lane. Imagine switching to another lane in order to get to your desired destination.

That is your goal right now--to get your body off the wrong road of toxic build-up to a cleansed road, from a road of tired organs to cleaned out revived organs.

Your job is to change the state of your body, by digging deep to uncover the root causes of your infertility.

Here are 10 things you can do immediately to get your body back on a healthy ready-to-conceive track:

1. Buy a juicer or a fruit/vegetable drink mixer. Learn as much as you can about making healthy vegetable and fruit drinks. Make this a daily part of your routine, whether it is simply juicing a bag of spinach or making a spinach/blueberry/flaxseed drink.

2. Find a reputable, licensed acupuncturist in your area and start going once, twice or even three times a week.

3. Visit a local health or nature food store and purchase a liver cleanse. You may want to do this more than once. This is to be done before you are in the midst of an IUI or IVF cycle.

4. Visit a supermarket and stock up on garlic, spinach, pumpkin seeds, sunflower seeds, kale, yams, and pineapple.

5. Schedule 20 minutes in your day to sit outside in the sunshine. Pick a place that feels comfortable—even if it is just putting a chair out in your front yard, a driveway or at a local park.

6. Find an excellent, highly reputable chiropractor in your area who is somewhat familiar with issues of infertility who can adjust your spine.

7. Start eating as much spinach and garlic as you can.

8. Get more sleep. Make sure your room is completely dark and get to bed earlier.

9. Stop drinking coffee and eating sugar.

10. Stop all trans fats that are in your diet. Cut down on white flour products too.

As always check with a physician before pursuing any course of treatment.

To begin:

• Start by having a complete physical: Go to your primary care physician and request a complete work-up.

You need to find out if you have:

• Gallstones

• Blood problems or disorders, such as anemia

• Ask for a complete work-up of your thyroid, liver and kidneys. This includes a thyroid stimulating hormone test and a comprehensive metabolic panel.

• Get tested for allergies, as you could be eating a food that weakens your body, such as gluten.

• Have your white blood cell count checked. This might help in determining if there is an undetected infection in your body.

The aim of the physical is to find out if there is an area in your body that has been overlooked, because one weak area can throw off the rest of the body.

• **Visit Your Dentist:** Get a complete dental check-up to be sure there are no lingering or untreated infections in your mouth.

Cleansing and Detoxifying Your Body

12 Cleanses To Help Restore Your Fertility

The next step in changing the state, or condition, of your body is cleansing and detoxifying. The importance of detoxifying your body should never be underestimated. In this chapter, we'll look at 12 cleanses that can help restore and maximize your fertility potential.

Please note: cleanses should be done before you start infertility medications or treatments, because you do not want them to interfere with medications or a pregnancy, if there is even a slight chance you could be pregnant. Cleansing can be compared to overturning and fertilizing the soil before planting the seed.

If you are just starting infertility treatments, you may want to choose just one or two cleanses, so as not to delay treatment.

If you've been trying to get pregnant for a long time with no success, you might want to consider doing various cleanses to strengthen your body.

Here are some cleanses to consider:

• A Liver Cleanse

Never never NEVER underestimate the importance of having your liver cleaned and detoxified. The liver is a highly influential organ that plays a key role in fertility and is one of the most important organs in your body. The liver governs approximately 500 metabolic processes and many studies have shown that the oestrogen receptors in the liver are critical for maintaining fertility.

I cannot say enough about the importance of having a clean, de-toxified liver in the quest to get pregnant.

An ineffective liver allows toxins to seep into the ovaries and endocrine system.

If your liver is congested, it cannot adequately remove toxins and fats from the body.

Instead, they will continue to recirculate through your system—causing hormonal disturbances and imbalances. It also means your ovaries will be flooded with toxic substances that your liver was suppose to clean—and your ovaries are the source of your eggs. These impurities will result in poor egg quality—all because your liver was too congested to do its job. So if you want to improve the quality of your eggs, make sure your liver is as clean and detoxified as possible.

Once the liver is cleansed, the entire endocrine and reproductive system becomes free of toxins and impurities, so they can begin functioning at a higher capacity.

What causes a sluggish, tired liver? Stress, poor diet, medication, toxins in the environment, low-quality food, coffee, sugar, white flour products and low quality drinking water, are among a few of the culprits. The older we get, the more our liver needs to be cleaned out because of the junk that we have taken into our body over the years.

A liver cleanse will help kick your body into high gear, increasing energy and vitality to all your organs.

Liver cleanses can be found online and at most health and natural food stores. You may want to do a 30-day cleanse more than once. Please note: A liver cleanse should never be done while you are taking infertility medications, as it could interfere with the effectiveness of the medication. It is something to do BEFORE you begin any infertility treatments or medication, and is never to be done if you could be pregnant.

In addition to a liver cleanse, here are some other ways to detoxify, cleanse and strengthen your liver:

• Milk thistle is a wonderful herb for cleansing the liver. Read the directions on the bottle carefully as to amounts taken.

• Lemon is a great liver cleanser. About 20 minutes before breakfast in the morning, squeeze the juice from one or two fresh lemons into some warm water and drink.

• Beets are excellent liver cleansers. You can eat them cooked or juice them. To juice beets, peel and cut into small wedges that can easily fit in your juicer. Juice the beets with some apple, spinach or kale.

• Chlorophyll is a highly esteemed liver cleanser.

• Artichokes are powerful liver protectors because they contain a flavonoid called silymarin, which is an antioxidant that protects the liver from toxicity.

• Foods that are good for your liver include: spirulina, garlic, carrots, romaine lettuce, apples, grapefruit, chicory, mustard greens, dandelion greens, avocados, walnuts, turmeric and parsley.

• Cabbage can also be juiced and is effective in cleaning the liver.

• Amino acids, derived from healthy sources of protein, are key to the liver working at maximum capacity. Foods that contain these amino acids include: nuts, such as pumpkin seeds, squash seeds and almonds; lean meats, eggs, and beans, such as lentils and garbanzo.

• In Chinese medicine, infertility is often linked to Liver chi stagnation, a result of stress, overwork, and the effects of coffee and alcohol. Irritability, headaches and frustration are just some of the physical and emotional symptoms of liver chi stagnation. Acupuncturists and herbalists can work on unblocking energy stagnation in the liver.

• According to Chinese medicine, emotional and lifestyle cures for liver stagnation include being assertive, making clear decisions and enjoying lots of fun, laughter and relaxation. Holding on to anger, feeling stuck and depression impair the liver by stagnating the energy. Letting go, moving on, and exercising control over one's life, can help in healing the liver.

• Heavy Metal Cleanse

Every day, we come into contact with heavy metals that can disrupt our fertility. As much as possible, you'll want to start paying attention to the metals you may be unintentionally bringing into your body through the products you use and your lifestyles choices. Cosmetics, drinking soda straight from a can, deodorants that contain aluminum, solvents in dry cleaning, exposure to radiation, all contain metals that can find their way into our body, causing metabolic disruptions in organs, such as our heart, brain, kidneys and liver.

Because heavy metals are so common in our world, most of us have them in our systems.

There are a variety of heavy metal cleanses available online and in health food stores. You may want to do this cleanse more than once. This is, however, a cleanse to be done before you start infertility treatments and medications.

Along with a heavy metal cleanse, here are some additional ways to cleanse your body of heavy metals:

• Garlic is known to help reduce metal levels in the body. It contains the antioxidant allicin. You can eat garlic raw, include it in your cooking or juice it. To juice, simply peel the garlic, juice, and drink combined with lemon juice and water. Have a big glass of water nearby to help reduce stomach discomfort.

• Milk thistle is an herb that can also help remove heavy metals from the liver.

• Cilantro is a powerful herb that is known for binding heavy metals and whisking them out of the body.

• Alpha Lipoic Acid and Gluthatione are powerful supplements for helping cells remove heavy metals from the body.

• Chlorella is a fresh water algae loaded with chlorophyll. Buy it in powder form and mix with water for fast absorption. It can also be taken in capsule or tablet form.

• A steam bath can help remove metals.

• Burdock is a potent blood purifier and can remove heavy metals from the body. It also helps purify the liver.

• Onions contain the antioxidant quercetin, which helps remove heavy metals from the body. Add to your salads daily or juice them.

• A Yeast Cleanse

Yeast, also known as candida, can impact your fertility by causing your internal vagina's flora to become unbalanced, making it difficult for sperm to reach the uterus.

Candida is a common yeast that lives in our gut, and an overgrowth of it can lead to leaky gut syndrome, which wreaks havoc with many of the body's systems, including the endocrine system, that plays a huge role in reproduction and fertility

Yeast can also impact estrogen levels in the body, causing thyroid problems and hormonal imbalances. Yeast problems can come from frequent or long-term use of antibiotics, birth control pills, or eating foods with a lot of sugar. Getting rid of yeast is an important step in rebalancing your body so it can heal itself.

Some ways to rid your body of yeast:

• Do a yeast or candida cleanse, that can be bought online, at health food store or nature food store.

• Acidophillus can help control candida.

• Flaxseed is known to help control yeast.

• Garlic is an enemy of yeast. Take garlic capsules, juice garlic and eat lots of raw garlic.

• Avoid sugar and white flour foods. These can include sugary juices, desserts, breads, crackers, pre-packaged meals, soda. Be alert to foods with hidden sugar, such as salad dressings or ketchup. Avoid alcohol, chocolate, cakes and carbonated beverages.

• Eat plain yogurt.

• Consider taking probiotics in a supplement form.

• Enzyme supplements are available that are made specifically to fight yeast.

• Replace your regular salt with Celtic salt or kosher salt.

• Adrenal Cleanse

Adrenal fatigue, also known as adrenal burn-out, impacts many women suffering with infertility. If you are having trouble getting pregnant, this could be one of the not-so-obvious and sometimes difficult to diagnose reasons behind your infertility.

The adrenals are a very important to your fertility because they are part of the endocrine system, which is responsible for producing and balancing more than 50 hormones in your body. When the adrenals are weak or not working at full capacity, the body's entire endocrine system and hormones can become imbalanced.

Adrenal burn-out occurs when the adrenals are stressed and pushed to the point where they begin producing excessive amounts of cortisol and adrenaline, which results in progesterone in the body producing too many stress hormones.

The adrenals become too sluggish, and then the other endocrine glands are not signaled to release their hormones, which results in the entire communication system in the endocrine glands breaking down.

Emotional trauma, living in a constant state of fight or flight, chemical toxins, lack of sleep, anxiety, stress, depression, poor diet, infections, and some prescription drugs, can all cause adrenal burn-out.

If the adrenals are exhausted, you may not produce enough progesterone, which is the pro-gestational hormone needed to get pregnant and carry a pregnancy to term.

Here are some ways to help strengthen your adrenals:

• Take a Vitamin C supplement. The adrenal gland uses vitamin C at a higher rate than other cells in the body.

• Don't let your blood sugar levels get too low. Eat regular meals and never skip breakfast. Keep your blood sugar levels normal by eating healthy foods throughout the day.

• Stop drinking coffee or drink no more than one cup of coffee a day. Caffeine depletes the body of B vitamins, which the adrenals need. Stop trying to energize and push your body by drinking another cup of coffee. Instead, eat fruits and vegetables that will provide your body with healthy forms of energy.

• Drink lots of high-quality water.

• Consider taking a Vitamin B complex, Vitamin E and an adrenal gland supplement.

• A high-quality liquid trace mineral supplement can help support the adrenal glands. Note: Although you may want to drastically reduce your intake of this supplement once you are pregnant, or consult with a doctor on the levels of minerals that are safe and healthy to take during pregnancy.

• Make lifestyle changes that reduce stress in your life. Do you need to change jobs? Relocate? Take a hard and honest look at the way you live your daily life. Start including more activities in your life that eliminate stress and reduce a fight-or-flight way of living. These include: deep breathing, massage, daily walks by a lake, ocean or in a beautiful park.

Consider more time for prayer, journal writing, and positive visualization.

• Foods that help adrenals include spinach, garlic, onions, green leafy vegetables and brown rice.

• Almonds and cashews, which are high in magnesium, are very healthy for the adrenal system.

• Eat more seeds, such as sunflower and pumpkin seeds.

• Avoid white flour products, soda, sugary fruit juices or anything that makes blood sugar levels rise rapidly.

• Alternative health therapies, such as applied kinesiology, myofascial release, and craniosacral therapy can restore a weakened adrenal system.

• Getting more sleep and better sleep can help restore the adrenal glands. So, go to bed earlier, preferably aim for a 9 to 10 o'clock bedtime, and try to stop all technology and electronic stimulation about an hour before bed for a better quality sleep.

• Sea salt, celtic salt or regular salt in moderate amounts can help the adrenal system provided that you don't suffer from high-blood pressure.

• Healthy fats like olive oil, coconut oil, ground flax seed or flax seed oil are excellent for burnt-out and exhausted adrenals.

• Adrenal exhaustion can sometimes be caused by hidden food allergies. Find out if you are allergic to wheat, corn or dairy products.

For the rest of the cleanses, which include a colon cleanse, kidney cleanse, parasite cleanse, uterine cleanse, blood cleanse, lymph system cleanse and thyroid cleanse, visit www.amazon.com to purchase Dancing Your Way to Fertility.

My Diary: Throughout this book, I will share my experience of infertility. This was the first essay I wrote at the start of my journey.

Today is my first day of writing a journal on my road to victory over infertility. I am writing this book for women like me who have been told that their eggs are too old, that our bodies are too old, weak, or damaged, that there is little hope. I am writing this book for women who feel that having a child is some type of impossible dream, that they are the victim of some pathologically cruel biological problem.

I am writing this book for women who, like me, dream of starting a family, but find the road long, cruel, uphill, and not always forgiving of slight mistakes and accumulated years.

I am 36 years old. Last week, a doctor that seemed very kind when I first met her told me that my eggs were the 'bottom of the barrel.' I have been seething with pain and engulfed in sadness ever since.

'Bottom of the barrel' the very image leaves me feeling hopeless. I cannot yell at her. I cannot criticize her. For if I do, the clinic may label me 'psychologically unfit' to undergo further infertility treatments. So I stay quiet. I watch my words. I must adhere to and accept as normal their warped and perverse idea that pulling hope away is truly in the best interest of the patient, when with all my heart I know that it is only hope and faith that will ultimately give me the baby I so desperately want. What kind of monsters are they? I so want to walk into that clinic, tell that monster doctor disguised as a kind, caring medical professional off, and never step foot in there again. But then what? I have no choice but to bite my tongue, and wait until it is my turn to walk in there with a beautiful baby and say, "hello, do you want to see what bottom of the barrel looks like?' That is when my victory will be complete.

For now, I wait and suffer and try to erase their hopeless images from my head.

In this book, I will recount my experience with infertility.

I will tell you now that this book will end with my successfully creating the family I dream of. I say this with confidence, for I believe God created us with a body that can heal and thrive and grow past illness, and that doctors do not understand the miracle of faith and the miracle of hope.

And for that doctor who tried to destroy my hope, I dedicate this book to you and anyone else who believes in stomping on a women's hope.

I don't always believe in being realistic—in putting my faith in only what I can see. Sometimes holding on to a dream takes being strong enough to push aside the skeptics, the cynics, the naysayers and delving into the world of hope--a world that takes a lot of strength to hold on to when everything around you is crumbling.

I begin this day by swimming. I am trying to get as healthy as possible. In the world of infertility, at 36, I am labeled old, but I don't feel old. Well, yes, maybe I do feel old. Withered inside at times. I just went through a harrowing IVF that ended with my becoming pregnant, only to lose the baby within two weeks of conception.

Cruel. That is how I feel right now about the past two weeks: cruel. They dubbed this pregnancy a chemical pregnancy, relegating it to something that almost didn't happen, didn't really happen, never existed. Thus was taken my right to feel sad or mourn, as it wasn't a pregnancy and it wasn't a miscarriage, but it was in a way, or is it? Nothing...dismiss it...mourning stamped invalid.

Most of all, I dedicate this book to God, who is the strength of my life. Without the privilege of prayer, I could not endure the hell of infertility. When the load was too heavy, it was only through prayer to God that I kept one foot in front of the other and kept trying.

So together, I begin this journey with you, a fellow infertility victim and survivor. I pray that we all see victory, in whatever form we wish it to come. For those of you wanting a child, I pray for your victory.

For those of you who have come to the point that adoption is a joyful option, I pray for you. I pray that we all can have the families we want and deserve, for family is a blessing and a gift, and all women deserve to receive this treasure of security, companionship, love and purpose.

To read other entries from my infertility diaries, you can purchase Dancing Your Way to Fertility or The Infertility Diaries at www.amazon.com.

Balancing Your Hormones and Improving the Quality of Your Eggs

• Balancing Your Hormones

If our hormones are not balanced, our fertility is compromised on every level. Our hormones, produced by our glands and tissues, are chemical communicators that deliver messages to our body. These messages are then released into our blood, where they travel to other tissues and send signals initiating various activities within our body and brain.

Hormones affect how we think and feel.

Our hormones are impacted by stress, fluid changes in the body, vitamin and mineral levels, infections, exposure to environmental toxins and body fat. Blood sugar imbalances, a toxic liver, folic acid deficiency, inflammation in the ovaries, breast and joints, and unhealthy gut flora can all be a result of unbalanced hormones.

Other symptoms of a hormonal imbalance can include insomnia, headaches, migraines, anxiety, foggy thinking, hot flashes, mood swings, thinning hair, bloating, rapid heartbeat, and allergies. Our hormones are impacted by stress, fluid changes in the body, vitamin and mineral levels, infection and exposure to environmental toxins and body fat.

It is important to support and strengthen the entire endocrine system. Hormones are coordinated by this system, which includes the hypothalamus, pituitary gland, adrenal gland, thyroid, parathyroid, pancreas, pineal gland, thymus and ovaries. The foods you eat, the stress levels you experience, the chemicals in your environment, all impact the endocrine system, and in turn, your hormones.

Progesterone is a key hormone in fertility and you want to do whatever you can to make sure you have adequate progesterone levels in your body.

Progesterone plays an important role in conception and maintaining a healthy pregnancy. It works to balance the effects of estrogen. It helps maintain the lining of the uterus, which makes it possible for a fertilized egg to attach and survive.

It also makes cervical mucous accessible to the sperm, preventing immune rejection of the developing baby and normalizes blood clotting. Progesterone is produced by the corpus luteum in the ovaries and by the adrenal glands.

One of the main causes of a progesterone defiency is too much estrogen in the body. Estrogen dominance is extremely dangerous to one's fertility. It can result from eating a lot of commercially raised meat and dairy products that contain large amounts of estrogen. Chemicals called xenoestrogens are often in these food sources and they mimic the hormone estrogen and disrupt the delicate balance between estrogen and progesterone. Other excess hormones and hormone-like substances found in our environment, food and water also impact progesterone levels in the body. Pollution, stress, processed foods, soy products, and endometriosis, can cause an overload of estrogen. Allergies like asthma, hives, dry eyes, weight gain, irregular periods, and foggy thinking are symptoms of estrogen dominance.

A low thyroid, recurrent early miscarriages, sleep disturbances, and heart palpitations, can sometimes be symptoms of progesterone deficiency.

Other hormones important to fertility include estradiol, or estrogen, that are produced by the follicles and corpus luteum, also known as the remnant egg sac in the ovaries. The luteinizing hormone, known as the LH surge, produced in the anterior pituitary gland, triggers ovulation and the development of the corpus luteum. It works in conjunction with the follicle stimulating hormone (FSH) that is also released and synthesized by the anterior pituitary gland. The FSH hormone regulates the reproductive process and signals the follicles in the ovary to begin maturing in preparation for ovulation.

Tests that can track your hormone levels include progesterone, estradiol, FSH, LH, prolactin, testosterone, sex hormone binding globulin, glucose tolerance test, thyroid panel and a blood lipid panel.

Here are some ways to balance and maintain healthy fertility hormone levels in your body:

• Reduce your exposure to xenohormones, which can be found in car exhaust, plastics, solvents, adhesives, pesticides, and emulsifiers found in soap and cosmetics and PCD's from industrial waste.

• Consider the herb Chaste Tree Berry, also known as Vitex Extract, that can balance hormones and strengthen the pituitary and ovary glands. This herb can correct hormonal communication in the body and hormonal problems at their source.

• Progesterone shots. You may want to talk to your doctor about progesterone shots if you had recurrent miscarriages or just want help maintaining your pregnancy. This is something to consider requesting if your doctor has not initiated it and if you exhibit the symptoms of a progesterone deficiency.

• Natural progesterone cream. Check with your doctor and discuss the amount to use.

• Vitamin B6 is known to help maintain optimal levels of progesterone and is key in progesterone production. Vitamin B also helps the liver break down estrogen. Food sources of Vitamin B6 can be found in walnuts, lean red meat, poultry, bananas, spinach, and potatoes.

• Turmeric, thyme and oregano are all considered helpful in raising progesterone levels.

• Vitamin C is known to considerably increase progesterone production.

• Zinc is key for producing adequate levels of progesterone in the body. That is because Zinc is a mineral that prompts the pituitary gland to release follicle stimulating hormones, which in turn promote ovulation and stimulate the ovaries to produce estrogen and progesterone.

Along with a zinc supplement, natural sources of zinc include lean red meats, wheat germ, chickpeas, pumpkin and squash seeds, watermelon and dark chocolate.

• Practice stress-reduction techniques, as stress can considerably reduce progesterone levels in the body.

• Do you have low cholesterol? This can mean you are not making enough pregnenolone, which is used to make progesterone.

• Are your adrenals healthy? They house DHEA that is essential to the production of progesterone. One way to improve your adrenal health is to improve your natural circadian rhythm and get more sleep.

• Maintain a healthy digestive tract. If you have a damaged digestive tract, you won't have the raw materials within your body to absorb the nutrients in your food that helps the body produce hormones.

• You may want to consider testing for parasites, candida, or pathogens which can impact your hormonal balance.

• Maca, a root vegetable in the radish family, can balance hormones and nourish and balance the endocrine system. It protects the body from stress damage. Maca is a nutritionally dense super food that contains high amounts of minerals, vitamins, enzymes and all of the essential amino acids. Maca also stimulates and nourishes the hypothalamus and pituitary glands, which are the "master glands" of the body. It is available in powder form or capsules,

• Coconut oil stimulates the thyroid and provides omega-3's that help balance hormones. Other healthy fats essential to hormone health include flax oil, evening primrose oil and olive oil.

• Magnesium is known to break down excessive estrogens in the system and assist in balancing hormones. Kelp and cashews are rich in magnesium. Other sources of magnesium include black beans, spinach, okra, watermelon seeds, sunflower, pumpkin seeds and squash seeds.

• Garlic is an important nutrient for the endocrine system.

• Ginkgo and ginseng help regulate hormones

• Consider supplements such as Vitamin C and Vitamin B.
• Getting more sleep helps balance hormones.

• Flaxseed contains lignans and fiber, which help remove excess estrogen from the body.

• Hormone imbalances can be a result of obesity. Fat cells can create hormonal imbalances. If you think you are overweight, consider trying to lose some of the weight to help your hormonal system.

• Red Clover, an herb, protects the body from xenohormones.

• Black Cohosh, an herb, is well-known for its effect on hormone functioning.

• Do a liver cleanse. The liver plays a key role in to hormonal balance. Milk thistle, dandelion leaf and burdock root are all potent liver cleansers.

• Royal jelly is rich in amino acids and contains acetylcholine, which is needed to transmit nerve messages from cell to cell.

• Ashwagandha root supports endocrine system function and helps to regulate hormones.

• Be aware of chemicals in your diet, water, and environment that can throw your hormones out of balance.

• Drink only filtered water. Avoid water with fluoride. Fluoride is known to weaken the thyroid, one of the key organs responsible for your hormones.

• Be aware of products that may contain aluminium, including deodorants, anti-perspirants, and cosmetics.

• Be careful of meats coated with nitrate salts.

• Do not eat foods from plastic containers. Whenever possible, use glass and stainless steel.

• Avoid vegetable oil, canola oil, soybean oil, margarine, shortening and other chemically altered fats.

• Drink whole milk, not skim milk

• Licorice is a hormone balancer.

• Natural sources of iodine can help regulate hormones. These include kelp, cranberries and strawberries.

• Improve indoor air-quality with plants.

• Limit caffeine.

• Other supplements to consider for hormonal balance include calcium, Vitamin E and grapeseed extract.

• Address your hormonal imbalance on the emotional level. Are you feeling trapped? Unloved? Stuck? Angry? Are you living in a way that is true to who you are? Let your body tell you why your hormones are imbalanced.

• Foods To Help Balance Hormones

• Pumpkin seeds and Brazil nuts.

• Avocados and acai

• Spinach, kale, parsley, broccoli, asparagus and other leafy greens.

• Sweet peppers.

• Pears and peaches are known to help regulate hormones. They are used often in traditional Chinese medicine.

• Shiitake and reishi mushrooms, chia seeds, seaweed and spirulina.

• Avocados block estrogen absorption and promote progesterone production.

How to Improve Your Egg Quality

Good news—you can improve the health and quality of your eggs.

In the past, we were told we were all born with a certain number of egg cells that run out as we age. We were led to believe that egg cells were the only cells in the body that did not regenerate, but instead were a finite number. We are finding out THIS IS JUST NOT TRUE. Recent research has shown that women can produce new eggs throughout their reproductive years.

You may have been told that your eggs are not healthy or that your eggs are too old.

Here's the great news: there is much you can do to enhance the health of your eggs.

It was commonly believed that the only factor that determined egg health and quality was age. Several new studies have shown that stress, hormones and environmental toxins all impact our egg health.

Your egg's health is a key cornerstone of a healthy fertility, because the health of your eggs can affect whether or not fertilization, implantation and ultimately a healthy pregnancy and birth will occur.

Here are some things you can do to improve your egg health:

• Coenzyme Q10: Coenzyme Q10 is an excellent way to improve the quality and energy within your eggs. In several studies, the supplement Coenzyme Q10 has been shown to improve egg quality. It boosts energy production in the oocytes, which are cells in the ovary. Providing additional energy in the form of Coenzyme Q10 is needed when there is decreased energy production in the ovaries due to aging.

It is also a source of fuel for the mitochondria, which produces energy within the cells and with age, can begin to weaken. Along with taking a Coenzyme Q10 supplement, natural sources of CoQ10 include almonds, spinach, sardines, broccoli, strawberries, and walnuts.

• Green Tea: Green Tea contains hypoxanthine which provides follicular fluid that helps eggs mature, along with polyphenols that are powerful antioxidants that prevent chromosomal abnormalities, and repair oxidative damage within the body. However, green tea can reduce the body's absorption of folic acid, so you may want to increase your dosage of folic acid at the same time.

• Start eating foods high in antioxidants that will protect your eggs from free radical damage. Free radicals can damage both the egg cell health and the cell's DNA. Foods high in antioxidants that can combat free radicals include blueberries, cranberries, garlic, Granny apples, artichokes, spinach, kale, broccoli, plums, walnuts, and oregano.

• Include Maca in your diet, which is a root-like cruciferous vegetable and the only plant known in the world that can grow and thrive at a high altitude in harsh weather. Maca contains 31 different minerals and 60 different phytonutrients. It nourishes the endocrine system, aids the pituitary, adrenal and thyroid glands, and helps balance hormones and increases energy and stamina in the body.

Maca controls estrogen levels in the body, which is very important because if estrogen levels are too high or low, it can prevent a woman from becoming pregnant or carrying full term. Excess estrogen levels can also cause progesterone levels to become low. Make sure that when you purchase Maca, it contains the root, not just leaves and stem. Once, you are pregnant, you need to stop Maca immediately—it is to be taken only to prepare your body to become pregnant.

To read more on improving your egg health, the entire copy of Dancing Your Way to Fertility can be purchased at www.amazon.com

Strengthening and Preparing Your Organs

As you prepare to be pregnant, it is important to strengthen the various organs in your body.

• Your Vagina

You want to make your vagina a welcoming environment. A healthy vagina produces healthy cervical mucus, a key to conception. Healthy bacteria in one's vagina can enhance fertility, while an acidic or unhealthy vagina can be a barrier to fertility. Medications, illness, excessive douching, severe emotional stress, or clothing that holds in body heat and moisture, can upset the balance of a healthy vagina. You want to help make your vagina a welcoming environment.

Here are some ways to promote a healthy vagina:

• Wear cotton underwear for good air flow. This prevents the development of damp conditions that promote yeast and unhealthy bacteria. Avoid underwear made from synthetic fabrics, silk, lace and other materials that don't breath freely.

• Do not use douches or feminine sprays that can wash out healthy bacteria that helps the vagina stay clean and infection-free. Avoid scented creams, scented pads, scented tampons and wipes.

• Go to a doctor to see if you have bacterial vaginosis, which is an overgrowth of bacteria inside your vagina and should be treated.

• Check to see if you have any vaginal abnormalities that can impact fertility, such as fusion of the labia or an imperforate hymen.

• It is important not to ignore yeast infections and vaginal infections, such as vulvovaginitis.

• Sexually transmitted diseases, such as Chlamydia and gonorrohea, need to be treated.

• When you wash your vagina, use hot water rather than strong soaps. If you choose to use soap, make sure you thoroughly rinse your vaginal area with warm water so no trace of soap is left behind. Using harsh soaps can lead to infection, and irritation.

• Eat garlic. It has properties that kill yeast.

• Do not use lubricants of any kind.

• Aim to make your vagina less acidic and more sperm friendly. Ideally, your pH range should be at 6.5 to 7.5. If your body is acidic, your cervical mucus will also be acidic, thus creating a hostile environment for sperm.

• Avoid vegetable oil.

• Avoid saliva.

• Avoid glycerin.

• Minimize your intake of sugar, alcohol and white flour products.

• The gut flora, or bacteria in your gut, colonize your vagina. Eat sufficient probiotics or yogurt with bifidus and acidophilus cultures. Yogurt has lactobacillus acidophilus, or "good bacteria." Avoid sugary yogurt.
• L-Arginine increase production of mucus during ovulation.

• Calcium helps the pH balance of the cervical mucus be less acidic and more sperm friendly.

• Grapeseed extract protects the sperm and helpsthe cervical mucus sperm be more sperm-friendly.

• Vitamin C increases the amount of water in your cervical mucus, thus helping produce more cervical mucus.

• Avoid foods that make your blood acidic, such as processed foods, red meat and hydrogenated oils.

• Evening Primrose Oil helps increase cervical mucus production.

• Red clover and Siberian ginseng also help support vaginal health.

• Ovaries

The ovaries rely on fat for fertility and hormonal balance. Vitamins A and E found in foods such as olive oil and avocados support reproductive health. The antioxidants found in fruits and vegetables, especially those with a deep orange color, are known to strengthen the ovaries. These include sweet potatoes, cantaloupe, oranges, orange bell peppers. Vitamin B6 is also important to ovarian health. If you are deficient in B6, your body may produce more estrogen than you need, which disrupts the menstrual cycle and can prevent your ovaries from releasing eggs on a consistent basis. Foods rich in Vitamin B6 include avocado, spinach, broccoli, beans and potatoes.

• Thyroid

Undiagnosed thyroid problems can sometimes be at the root cause of infertility or recurrent miscarriages. To start, visit your primary care doctor and have your thyroid tested to find out the amount of the thyroid hormone your thyroid is secreting. Request a thyroid stimulating hormone test (TSH) with the full panel of thyroid levels, including thyroid antibodies and thyroxine. Ask for the numerical result for the TSH level. Some doctors believe that if a woman has a TSH level higher than 2.0, it may indicate that she will have problems getting pregnant.

Hypothyroidism, or an underactive thyroid, and hyperthyroidism, known as over-active thyroid, are sometimes pinpointed as the cause of infertility.

Both hypothyroidism and hyperthyroidism can cause imbalances which impact your ovaries.

The ovaries are very sensitive to changes in thyroid levels and even seemingly small declines in thyroid levels can adversely impact ovarian function. Some symptoms of a thyroid dysfunction include cold hands and feet, weight gain and depression.

If you have an underactive thyroid, it means your thyroid gland doesn't produce enough of certain hormones. Low levels of thyroid hormones can interfere with the release of eggs from your ovaries.

That's because the hypothalamus and pituitary glands can sometimes sense an underactive thyroid gland and try to kick things back to normal by increasing the levels of hormones in the body.
 Low levels of the thyroid hormone can interfere with ovulation, which impairs fertility.

Along with being treated by a doctor who specializes in thyroid problems, here are some other things you can do to help your thyroid condition:

• Eat foods high in vitamin A, such as yellow vegetables and dark green vegetables.

• Foods that contain iodine nurture the thyroid, such as kelp and seaweed. Seaweed can be added to soups, salads or just eaten plain. Other foods rich in iodine include: asparagus, bananas, carrots, garlic, onions, spinach, and tomatoes.

• Coconut oil is known to be excellent for boosting thyroid function.

• Foods rich in zinc nourish the thyroid, such as oatmeal, chicken and spinach.

• Raisins are rich in copper, which help the body produce thyroid hormones.

• Soy should not be eaten at this time, because soy can interfere with thyroid hormones.

• The amino acid Tyrosine, found in beef and chicken, help support the thyroid.

• Beet tops, leafy greens, and parsley are helpful in supporting thyroid function.

• Dark green leafy vegetables that are rich in minerals also boost the thyroid.

• Foods to avoid include cauliflower, brussel sprouts, canola oil, soy, peanuts, cabbage and kale, which have goitrogens that are high in sulfur have been known to impede thyroid gland function. A note of caution here, however, those with an overactive thyroid may find these foods helpful. It is recommended you meet with a physician or nutritionist to discuss which foods are best for you, depending on your thyroid condition.

• Avoid coffee, caffeine products and excessive amounts of alcohol.

• Keep your blood sugar levels steady, as fluctuating blood sugar levels can negatively impact the thyroid.

• Avoid artificial sweeteners, such as aspartame.

• Include a good quality sea salt or Celtic salt in your diet, instead of white table salt.

• For an underactive thyroid, consider foods like sea kelp, chicken, dates, molasses, and parsley.

• Reduce your intake of sugar as much as you can.

• Alternative therapies that can help the thyroid include acupuncture and lymph drainage massage, in which the thyroid and lymphatic system are massaged so as to loosen any blocks.

• Avoid drinking out of plastic and soda cans. Instead, drink only out of glass, stainless steel or BPA free plastic bottles.

• Include lots of natural fats in your diet, such as olive oil, flaxseed and avocados.

Vitamin and mineral supplements considered helpful to thyroid function include:

• B-complex

• Vitamin C

• Omega 3s that are found in fish, flaxseed and walnuts, which are the building blocks for the hormones that control immune function and cell growth.

• A multi-mineral formula in liquid form, since minerals are key to glandular health.

• Calcium/magnesium are also known to help the metabolic process.

• High-quality natural thyroid supplements. Note: you may want to seek the advice of a well-trained nutritionist on what type of supplements are appropriate for those who are trying to get pregnant, and what dosage is appropriate once you are pregnant or on infertility medications.

• You might want to consider a glutathione supplement and include in your diet foods that contain glutathione, such as asparagus, broccoli, peaches, spinach, garlic and grapefruit.

• Pay attention to your food allergies and sensitivies.

• Reduce gluten in your diet or if you can, go entirely gluten free.

• Take a probiotic, because for the thyroid to be healthy and function well, it needs and depends on having a sufficient supply of healthy gut bacteria.

• Pay attention to adrenal burn-out or fatigue, because there is a strong connection between the thyroid and adrenal glands.

Think of the thyroid and adrenals as Frick and Frack—if you have a problem with hypothyroidism, you are probably suffering with some level of adrenal fatigue or burn-out too.

• Include seaweed in your diet.

• Avoid excessive forms of radiation if you can.

• Do a heavy metal cleanse. Heavy metal exposure is sometimes linked to thyroid problems. In addition to a heavy metal cleanse, begin eating or juicing garlic and cilantro, and include such as taking Milk Thistle, turmeric and chlorella in your diet.

• Eat more foods that contain selenium, such as salmon, sunflower seeds, onions and brazil nuts.

• Stress and emotional traumas, such as a job loss or marital problems, can weaken thyroid function. Explore creative ways to reduce stress, such as joining a chorus, taking gentle walks in a beautiful area, or take a painting or drawing class. Deep breath.

• The thyroid gland is located in the throat, the center of our communication with the world. Holistic practitioners often view low thyroid function as a result of a blocked throat chakra, a result of feeling like you can't speak your truth. It is important to learn new and creative ways of finding and using your voice, such as singing, writing and creating art. Stop 'swallowing' your feelings. Speak your truth instead. Create an expression center in your home, where you feel safe to freely say what you want to say and let your deepest feelings be known.

• Avoid drinking tap water.

• Do not use non-stick cookware.

• Stop using perfume for now, especially in the neck area.

• Eat foods that contain tyrosine, an amino acid the body needs to manufacture thyroid hormones, such as avocados, almonds, bananas, pumpkin seeds and lentils.

• Include more sea vegetables in your diet, such as kelp and kelp granules that can be sprinkled over your salads.

• Stay outside in the sunshine at least 20 minutes a day.

• Evening primrose oil is rich in amino acids which nourish the thyroid gland.

• Consider taking the herbs Nettle and Bladder Wrack.

• Discontinue using deodorants and body lotions that contain parabens, chlorates and pesticides.

To learn more about strengthening your organs, including your spleen and digestive system, pituitary gland, hypothalamus and thymus, pineal gland and pancreas, visit www.amazon.com to purchase Dancing Your Way to Fertility.

Important Ways To Enhance and Strengthen Your Fertility

• Start Making Vegetable Based Drinks Daily

If you want to cleanse and strengthen your body, by all means go out and buy a juicer or some type of bullet and start making vegetable based drinks on a daily basis. Do it today! Now! As soon as possible! This can change your body in a very big way. Making vegetable drinks is a wonderful and effective way to cleanse, alkalize and strengthen the body—three things you need to do to maximize your chances of getting pregnant.

When you make vegetable drinks, you are putting live food into your body. Many of the nutrients in foods are destroyed by cooking, so when you juice or blend vegetables, you are consuming these nutrients in an undisturbed form. It is one of the easiest, fastest ways to assimilate more nutrients into the body. Fresh, whole foods build healthy cells.

One of the health benefits of vegetable drinks is that it allows cellular cleansing on a deep level. When you are trying to fix an imbalance in the body, large amounts of fruits and vegetables can significantly help the body heal.

Making vegetable drinks helps your body become more alkaline, instead of acidic, which is a great booster in promoting fertility. Juicing will also give your body enhanced vitality.

Have I said enough about the power of daily vegetable drinks? Make yourself a healthy vegetable drink each day and you will feel and see almost immediately what a great healer and fertility enhancer it is.

To start, buy a juicer or bullet that is easy to handle, easy to clean and that you don't find intimidating.

There are lots of good ones on the market.

A side note here: making vegetable drinks does not have to be overly time-consuming and complicated. If some of the recipes call for too many ingredients and overwhelm you, make vegetable drinks with one or two ingredients. Spinach and blueberries, spinach, flaxseed and blueberries, kale and strawberries, are just a few.

For me, a bag of spinach and some blueberries juiced each morning, or some garlic and lemon is often enough to put my body on the right track. Parsley, beets, kale can also be juiced alone. If you find eating fruit easy, I would stick to juicing vegetables that you might not normally consume as often. Many people like a spinach/apple combination that is also easy, quick and very effective.

Some juicing suggestions include:

• Garlic. I know, I know, it sounds horrible, but it really isn't. Peel a few cloves of garlic and juice. Then combine the garlic juice with the juice of one or two squeezed lemons. Then pour in lots of water. I usually drink mine slowly. I have a jug of water ready, because if you start to feel sick from the garlic, slugging down lots of water helps ease the nausea. Garlic does great and wondrous things for the body—so start drinking. I promise—it is not as bad as it sounds!)

Some nutritionists have suggested that garlic can also help prevent miscarriages and enhance both male and female fertility.

• Juice spinach for heightened doses of folic acid. Spinach is one of the vegetables I would recommend juicing almost daily. There are so many health benefits to spinach. Some people like to juice spinach with apples, or with other greens. Find the combination you like.

• Along with spinach, beets, asparagus, garlic and kale are considered among the best vegetables for treating infertility. Pineapple, strawberries and oranges are considered among the best fruits for enhanced fertility. Create vegetable/fruit drinks with these combinations.

• Juice kale, chicory, romaine lettuce, parsley.

• Some vegetables to avoid include celery. It is recommended not to juice celery while pregnant or trying to get pregnant.

• Carrots and beets is a mixture that is very healthy for the liver. Carrots provide huge amounts of Vitamin A to the body in a natural form, which is important because Vitamin A deficiency can prevent eggs from properly maturing.

• Other juice combinations can include:
-beet/carrot/radish/
-spinach/apple
-carrot/apple,parsley
-kale/spinach/apple
-ginger/apple
-apple/pear.
-Pineapple/strawberry/spinach
-Cucumber/spinach/celery/apple
-Kale/spinach/apple/carrot
-Apple/carrot/pineapple/celery/lemon
-Parsley/kale
-Kale/spinach/cabbage/mint
-Kale, pineapple and ginger detox.
-Pineapple, lemon and pomegranate
-Fennel, garlic and cabbage

• Other fruits and vegetables that can be juiced and are known to help fertility include red peppers, dark green leaf lettuce, onions, cabbage, broccoli and dark leafy greens.

• You can also add chia seeds, maca, flaxseeds, spirulina, cayenne pepper, and turmeric to your drinks.

• Increase Circulation to Your Reproductive System

Begin to do self-massage. Since many of us hold stress in our stomach, massaging your stomach can help reduce stress and help your digestion. Do not do massage if there is a possibility you could be pregnant.
If you are not pregnant, massage your liver, kidney, and ovaries.
Put your legs up against a wall to increase blood circulation to the pelvis and ovaries. You can also increase circulation to your reproductive system by brushing your skin to remove toxins. Or take a very hot shower for five minutes, and then follow with cold water for 30 seconds. Green grapes can also improve circulation. Stretch often. Drinking lemon, cayenne pepper and apple cider vinegar can also increase circulation.

• Restore Good Bacteria In Your Body

One way to become more fertile is to restore good bacteria in your body.

Eating yogurt that has little to no sugar, and contains live active cultures is one way to do this. Avoid or reduce your intake of sugar and caffeine. Olive oil and avocados are known to help restore good bacteria in the body.

Foods high in good bacteria include apples, beets and sour cream.

Eat a diet low in white flour or gluten products.

Start taking a high-quality probiotic supplement.

To learn more about enhancing your fertility, including information on exercise, medications, electromagnetic energy, sleep, chemicals in the environment, sunlight, water, deep breathing and cervical mucous, Dancing Your Way to Fertility can be purchased at www.amazon.com

Conditions That Might Be Threatening Your Fertility

Some of these conditions could be among the causes of your infertility.

• Do You Have An Iron Deficiency?

Some studies have found a link between low iron intake and infertility. Low iron, or anemia, can increase the body's risk for being unable to produce healthy eggs. This is because a lack of iron can cause anovulation, or lack of ovulation and in turn, poor egg health. Being low in iron can cause eggs stored in the ovaries to be weak and unviable.

A lack of iron in the body also results in an insufficient number of red blood cells, which are responsible for delivering oxygen to the ovaries and uterus. Ask your physician for a test to see if you are anemic or low in iron. You may want to consider taking a high-quality iron supplement, either in capsule or liquid form, or a multivitamin that has iron in it. Some studies have shown that it is best to take a vegetable based iron, rather than animal based.

• Eat more foods high in iron. These include spinach, beets, molasses, pumpkin seeds, asparagus.

Other iron rich foods include:

• Kale, broccoli, lean red meat, asparagus, parsley, kidney beans, lentils, apricots, and chicken.

• When you get pregnant, make sure your iron levels are sufficient throughout your pregnancy.

• Select an iron supplement that includes nutrients that help iron absorption, which are B12 (folic acid) and Vitamin C.

• Consider Your Weight

Being overweight can cause your body to produce excess insulin, which stimulates the ovaries to produce testosterone male-like hormones. Being overweight can also cause hormonal irregularities and increase one's risk of miscarriage. So if you are overweight, do what you can do lose weight.

When I was trying to get pregnant for a second time, I was told that if I lost weight, my chances for conception would improve significantly. So I went to Friendly's, enjoyed a big five-scoop sundae with lots of hot fudge, and then I joined Weight Watchers. Over the course of seven months, I lost almost 50 pounds. I do believe this helped in my ultimately getting pregnant.

My diet consisted of a lean turkey meat sandwich with healthy bread and mustard, instead of mayonnaise. I also ate a lot of bowls of romaine lettuce and parsley as snacks at work. I was sometimes called a 'rabbit' by my co-workers, and my nightly treat was sugar free, fat free pudding, although I stopped eating this the closer I got to the IVF procedure. I also ate a lot of Weight Watcher's garden vegetable soup.

Cut down on white flour products, sugary juices, sodas and sugar. Write down everything you eat each day. Prepare snacks of cut and washed fruits and vegetables ahead of time each night, so you don't slip during the day. Find a support group or therapist to help if you relied on food to cope with emotional needs, such as loneliness or frustration. Do one thing each day to lose weight.

• Is Your Body's Energy Off Track?

Keeping the energy flow in your body on track is important to good health. In Chinese medicine, infertility is seen as an imbalance of the body's energy levels and that to heal one's infertility it is important to find the imbalances in the body, and then balance the body's organs, hormones, and energy systems.

Restoring balance and getting the body back on track can be done through improved diet, cleansing and detoxifying, releasing stress, and getting consistent acupuncture treatments, along with other holistic methods.

• Do You Have A Tooth or Gum Infection?

Go to your dentist for a thorough cleaning and check-up. A problem with your teeth can weaken the whole body. Do you have any infected teeth? Do you have any cavities that need to be filled? Excessive plaque that needs to be cleaned? Do you need a root canal or a crown? Is there a hidden infection in your teeth that needs to be addressed? It is important that you make sure all infections in your teeth are cleared up and when you begin infertility treatments.

• Is Your Back or Spine Out of Alignment?

Do not underestimate the role your spine plays in your body's mechanics. There are studies that have shown a link between spinal adjustments and increased fertility, because the nerves to the reproductive system run through the spine. When the back is misaligned, the nerves can misfire and cause a hormone imbalance. Getting your spine and body in alignment can help all your organs function at a higher level and increase your energy flow.

Consider finding an experienced chiropractor and getting an adjustment. A chiropractor can identify spinal distortions, also called subluxations, that once corrected can improve infertility.

If your spine is properly aligned, your nervous system will have a better chance of working at maximum capacity. Think of what happens when your car is properly aligned--your wheels last longer and other parts of your car work better because they are not having to compensate for an unaligned car. The body works in much the same way.

If your spine is out of alignment, your legs or hips can also be off and weaken the energy and flow in your lower body.

Infections can live in your spine, and if your spine has an infection, it can impact the way your organs communicate with one another.

• Is Your Body Too Acidic?

When you are trying to get pregnant, one of your goals should be to make the environment within your body as alkaline as possible.

 Imagine preparing soil for planting—the healthier the soil is, the better chance the seed will have to survive.

More than ever before, your body needs to be alkaline, not acidic. Poor eating habits, lack of exercise, and toxic elements in the environment, can cause your body to become acidic.

Eating lots of acidic foods result in cervical mucus that is an acidic, which is a hostile environment for sperm. Sperm needs an alkaline environment to survive.

You can test the alkaline/acid in your body with pH strips.

To alkalize your body, start your day by drinking a large glass of water with a freshly squeezed lemon.

Foods that alkalize the body include watermelon, apple cider vinegar, artichokes, asparagus, unsalted almonds, coconut oil, lettuce, broccoli, spinach and olive oil.

Chew your food thoroughly.

Foods that help promote an alkaline environment in the body include parsley, garlic, barley grass, green beans, lima beans, zucchini, lemon, beets, asparagus, cabbage, kale, onions, spirulina, flax seeds, sea vegetables, dandelion root, green tea, pumpkin seeds, brussel sprouts. spinach, broccoli, and green leafy vegetables. Figs, apples, grapes, bananas, watermelon, wheatgrass and barley grass are alkaline producing foods.

Meat, bread, carbonated drinks, coffee, sugar, fast foods, sodas, muffins, waffles, pancakes, bacon, sausage often promote high levels of yeast and fungi in the body, leading to higher acid levels.

Allergies, arthritis, acne, heart attacks, and weight problems are often linked to an improper pH balance, or acid, in the body.

 If your body is alkalized, you are creating an internal environment conducive to pregnancy.

For more on conditions that could cause infertility, such as infections, allergies, celiac disease and body temperature, Dancing Your Way to Fertility can be purchased on amazon.com.

Holistic and Alternative Health Treatments To Consider

• Acupuncture

Without a doubt, acupuncture has been shown to help heal infertility and is one of the best and most effective ways to strengthen your reproductive system.

Begin acupuncture treatments as soon as possible. Now! Today! Immediately! Acupuncture is a wonderful and life changing way to get to the root of some of your fertility problems. Numerous studies have shown that acupuncture dramatically helps infertile couples get pregnant and increases the success rate of IVF and other assisted reproductive technologies.

Acupuncture improves ovarian function, hormonal balance, and helps regulate the chemical pathways in the ovaries, pituitary gland and hypothalamus.

Some studies have shown that acupuncture increases your egg health, and keep eggs healthier than they would normally be without treatment.

Acupuncture also increases blood flow to the ovaries and the uterus, which is very important, because enhanced blood flow can help thicken the lining of the uterus.

Acupuncture also helps correct problems in the endocrine system, which includes the thyroid and hypothalamus, key organs in fertility. Acupuncture can strengthen the liver and kidneys, and help activate the brain to release hormones that stimulate the ovaries, adrenal glands and other organs involved in reproduction.

Acupuncture can moves the body over from a track of disease and dysfunction to a track of health.

It enhances your energy, removes energy blocks in the body, and shifts energy back on to proper pathways. If there is a blockage in your energy pathway, acupuncture can clear the blockages and allow energy to flow smoothly. By rerouting blocked energy, acupuncture restores the proper balance of yin and yang in the body.

Begin the process of acupuncture and commit to it. To see the benefits of acupuncture takes time and patience. Don't expect to go just once or twice and suddenly have your energy in perfect tune. It takes consistency, but if you stay on track with your weekly treatments, you will eventually see great results.

Try to find someone who has some experience treating infertility patients, but if you can't, that is fine too. If possible, try to go at least twice a week. If you can afford it, go three or four times or as many times as you can.

If money is an issue, you may want to talk with your acupuncturist about getting treatments at a reduced rate. They may be open to giving you a discount if you commit to a certain number of appointments each month, or if you offer to pay up front for five to ten or more appointments at once. Some acupuncturists may discount the treatments for bulk payments. Or some might give you a discount if they know your situation and know you are going to be a long-term customer. In some areas, there are also community acupuncture clinics, also known as group acupuncture, that offer a sliding scale for treatments and are significantly less expensive than one-on-one appointments.

The more acupuncture appointments you can do, the better. Once, during the week I had an IUI scheduled, I went three times to help me conceive, which I ended up doing successfully.

Up until the actual time that you do an IUI or IVF, you can continue acupuncture. There is some disagreement as to whether or not acupuncture should be done once you are pregnant. That is a personal opinion and should be researched and discussed with your acupuncturist. I reserved this wonderful treatment for pre-pregnancy preparation only.

If you have an upcoming IVF or IUI, do acupuncture a few times before the procedure.

Bottom line is: you will dramatically increase your chances of if you do acupuncture on a weekly, or preferably, twice weekly basis, for a period of several months.

• Bio Cleanse

An ionic food bath, also known as a bio cleanse ionic detox foot bath, pulls toxins out of the body through the feet. Positive and negative ions are emitted by the ionic foot bath machine, and helps the body rebalance and eliminate toxins in the kidneys, bowel, liver and skin.

A holistic practitioner in your area may have this machine that can remove yeast, parasites, and heavy metals from your liver, kidneys and muscles.

This should only be done as a preparation for infertility treatments, and not once you have started infertility medication or treatments, such as an IUI or IVF. Do not do this if there is any chance you are pregnant. Nor is it safe for anyone with an organ transplant, pacemaker or epilepsy.

• Lymphatic Massage or Manual Lymphatic Drainage

This is a gentle massage that encourages the natural drainage of the lymph from the tissues in the body.

This type of massage is very helpful to your lymph system and is an excellent way to detoxify before an IVF or other types of fertility treatments. Stimulating the lymphatic system helps to drain swollen tissues, enhances the body's immune system, and helps the body's natural waste removal system.

• Applied Kinesiology

Applied kinesiology can provide you with some incredible emotional healing from trauma or sadness trapped in your body.

Our emotions have a physical component and can be energetically trapped in our body, impacting not only our emotional self, but our physical self too.

Sometimes, an event or experience can be so painful, that the emotional trauma of it physically lodges itself permanently in the body. This explains why some memories, betrayals, and traumas can feel so recent decades after they occurred, even when we try to let go and forget them.

In applied kinesiology, a chiropractor or holistic practitioner will use what is referred to a "the gun" or activator to release trauma and emotional pain in your body.

One way to help release trapped traumas in your body is to write a list of all the people, experiences, and events in your life that have hurt you. Give the kinesiologist this list, and ask them to muscle test and locate where these memories have physicall lodged themselves in your body. Once found, the kinesiologist can activate the "gun" to release or free these emotional energy blocks in your body. Once these traumas leave your body, you'll find yourself feeling better, both emotionally and physically. Your body will no longer be weighed down by intensely negative emotions that do impact your organs and entire body system.

Vitamins and Other Supplements that Can Help Prepare Your Body for Pregnancy

Start with a high-quality prenatal vitamin and a high-quality mineral supplement. If possible, see a reputable nutritionist or holistic health practitioner to start a balanced vitamin and herb regime.

Remember: some vitamins, herbs and supplements need to be stopped the moment you could be pregnant—some are for pre-pregnancy preparation only, and not safe once you have conceived. Other vitamins and herbs should not be taken at the same time you are taking infertility medications.

• A High-Quality Pre-Natal Vitamin

It is most important to start taking a pre-natal vitamin before you are pregnant to give your body the nutrients it needs.

• Omega-3

Some people consider Omega-3 a key part of a fertility health regimen. Omega-3 fats help fertility by regulating hormones, increasing cervical mucus, promoting ovulation and improving the overall quality of the uterus by increasing blood flow to the reproductive organs.

Omega-3 supplements also boost the immune system and reduce natural killer cells that can prevent the embryo's implantation in the uterus.

• Coenzyme 10

This is a supplement both you and your husband should consider taking—and be a supplement that you might consider your new best fertility friend! Recent studies have shown that Co-enzyme Q10 can actually help improve egg quality in older women and improve fertilization rates because it corrects the energy which impacts the division of chromosomes during fertilization.

It can improve the quantity and quality of your eggs, which is key to beating infertility. It is a major cellular antioxidant and can be considered giving your body a high grade fuel to up your cellular energy production process and protect your body from DNA damage. Ubiquinol, the active form of Coenzyme Q10, has demonstrated the ability to improve mitochondrial energy production in aged eggs.

Other studies have shown that it also helps improve sperm density and motility in men. This supplement has been shown to improve the rates of conception and live birth in women who are taking it.

• Folic Acid

You should begin taking folic acid long before you are pregnant in order to build it up in your system. The recommended dosages before pregnancy range from 400 mcg to 600 mcg. When I was trying to conceive, I opted for a higher dose of folic acid.

• Evening Primrose Oil

This oil is known to help produce fertile quality cervical fluid. This should only be taken BEFORE you are pregnant. STOP taking once if there is even a slight chance you could be pregnant. It aids in conception, but is not be taken at all during pregnancy.

• B complex

B6 balances hormone levels and improves low progesterone levels of women affected by luteal phase defect. B12 enhances ovulation and improves the inner lining of the uterus.

For more information on vitamins, the entire version of Dancing Your Way to Fertility can be purchased at www.amazon.com.

Powerful Foods To Help Cure Your Infertility

When working towards healing from infertility, never for one moment underestimate the power of the foods you eat.

Right now, this moment, you need to begin seeing everything you eat and drink as either a potential healer of your infertility or a potential destroyer of your fertility.

The foods you eat right now could mean the difference between getting pregnant and not getting pregnant. This is how important the food component of your fertility journey is.

Do not be fooled into thinking that you can drink lots of coffee, eat white flour products, sugar, and processed, fast-foods and it won't impact your body's ability to conceive.

Yes, there are some women who can live off fast food and still get pregnant whenever they choose—but there are also millions of women whose fertility is being stolen by the foods they eat.

To prepare for pregnancy, it is key that you plan, choose and decide to eat as healthy as possible to maximize your body's ability to have a baby.

Don't be trapped into thinking that you can eat the way you've always eaten and still heal your body.

If getting pregnant is not coming easily to you, you need to change your eating habits and let go of archaic ideas about food that could be holding your body back.

Every time you are tempted by that chocolate bar in the vending machine at work, or a cup of coffee, or a cracker with lots of hydrogenated oil, remind yourself that chocolate bar, or that cup of coffee, or that cracker, could be what ultimately prevents you from having a baby.

If you think a bagel, cream cheese and coffee is a healthy way to start to the day, think again.

It is simple: what you eat can make you weak or make you strong. The right foods can heal your infertility and the wrong ones can rob you of your right to be a mother.

Here are some tips that will help you use food as a way to heal your infertility and prepare your body for pregnancy:

To start:

• Stop Or Reduce Your Coffee Consumption

Do you drink coffee? You need to consider stopping. As much as you can, preferably stop all coffee. If you can't stop, drink no more than a half a cup to a cup a day. That's it. Ideally, do everything you can to say goodbye to coffee for now. Coffee is an enemy of your fertility. Every time you are tempted to drink coffee, remind yourself that this cup of coffee could rob you of the ability to give birth to children. Get rid of all caffeine products in your life. Extreme, maybe, but coffee can weaken key organs, such as the liver, and right now, you need to stack the odds in your favor.

Some studies have shown that women who drink high amounts of coffee take up to three times longer to conceive, and even small amounts of coffee can hamper fertility.

To cope with the lack of coffee in your life, you may need to go to bed earlier and eat healthier to compensate for the energy the coffee gave you to get through the day. Coffee cannot be your fuel or main source of energy anymore. Your energy has to come from healthy foods, vitamins, juices, exercise and other genuinely healthy energy-producing sources.

As you detoxify and strengthen your body, your energy will increase and come from your inner core of health—not coffee, an imposter who pretends to hand you energy, but ultimately steals it. Say goodbye to coffee and hello to food sources that genuinely fuel you.

• Eliminate Most Sugars

Do you eat lots of sweets? Realize that donuts, candy, cake, and other foods with sugar weaken your body and can prevent you from becoming pregnant.

Sugar puts your body in a diseased, acidic state. Sugar can cause hormone imbalances, vitamin deficiencies, high insulin levels, and a compromised immune system. While an occasional sweet is okay, overall you'll want to drastically reduce the sugar in your life.
It can be hard to quit eating all sweets entirely. Many of us have sugar cravings, but overall you want to drastically reduce the amount of sugar you consume.

You'll also need to be be aware and carefully examine the foods you eat that may have hidden sugars in them. Read labels carefully as sugar content varies by brand. Always remember: if its packaged, there is a chance it might have sugar in it.

Foods you need to be aware of for potential sugar content include:

- Yogurt
- Cereals
- Canned vegetables
- Canned soups
- Breakfast bars
- Salad dressing
- Condiments
- White flour products.
- Breads and rolls
- Juices
- Fast foods
- Barbecue sauce
- Soda
- Spaghetti sauce
- Energy drinks
- Dried fruit
- Crackers

• Products that list ingredients such as, dextrose, fructose, corn syrup, high-fructose corn syrup, fruit juice concentrate, lactose, sorbitol, xylitol, maltodetrin and turbinado sugar, polydextrose, mannitol, and turbinado sugar. Ingredients ending in 'ose' is often a likely form of sugar.
• Oatmeal
• Protein bars
• Ice tea
• Ketchup
• Frozen meal entrees, even diet ones
• Syrups
• Jelly and jams
• Fruit juice concentrate
• Bouillon cubes
• Bacon
• Luncheon meats

• Consider Reducing Hydrogenated Oils, Also Known As Trans Fats

Another category of food you need to consider cutting from your diet entirely are foods made with hydrogenated oils, also known as trans fats. Several studies have shown that women with fertility problems eat more trans fats or hydrogenated oils than fertile women. Hydrogenated oil is a man-made food substance used widely throughout the food industry because it lengthens the shelf life of many foods and is cost effective.

Trans fats interfere with the metabolic processes in the body, because they take the place of essential fatty acids that perform critical functions. Trans fats clog up the space that natural fats should occupy, making it difficult for essential nutrients to pass in and out of the cells. Bodily functions are altered by these artificial molecules that enter the system.
Various studies have shown that women who eat a diet high in hydrogenated oils are at increased risk for developing endometriosis.

The World Health Organization has tried to outlaw trans fats for decades.

Some say trans fats work against the body, because they cause a cell-by-cell failure that destroys the flexibility of healthy cell membranes—basically tearing the body down from the inside out.

Trans fats increase bad cholesterol, block production of chemicals that combat inflammation and benefit the body's hormonal and nervous systems. Trans fats are also linked to heart disease, stroke and diabetes.

They interfere with the absorption of essential fatty acids and DHA, and weaken cell walls and compromise cellular structure.

That means, if you are trying to get pregnant, you need to dramatically reduce eating foods made with hydrogenated oils, corn oil, vegetable oil, transfats and corn syrup.

Be sure to read food labels carefully so you are aware of what products contain hydrogenated oils.

Fast food restaurants often serve a lot of foods loaded with hydrogenated oils. Cake, pancake, biscuit, and cookie mixes are usually made with hydrogenated oils.

Diet foods that promise 'no fat' often have hydrogenated oils.

Labels that say partially hydrogenated, or hydrogenated, contain trans fats. Even foods that promise to be trans fat free may contain up to 0.5 grams of partially hydrogenated oil, a source of trans fats.

Remember that if you see the word 'hydrogenated' or partially hydrogenated, it means it contains a trans fat. Hydrogenated oils are also trans fats, and that includes hydrogenated coconut or soybean oil.

Read labels carefully because hydrogenated oil content can vary by brand.

Begin to replace hydrogenated oils with healthy oils your body needs, such as olive oil, coconut oil and flax seed oil.

It is best to avoid as many pre-packaged foods that you can at this time. Foods to be aware of can include:

- Commercially baked cakes, cookies, muffins, pies, donuts
- Crackers
- Peanut butter
- Frozen meals
- Frozen bakery items
- French fries
- Whipped toppings
- Margarines
- Shortening
- Cake frosting
- Taco shells
- Microwave popcorn
- Breakfast cereals
- Corn chips and potato chips
- Frozen pizzas and frozen burritos
- Low-fat ice creams
- Pre-made noodle soups and soup mixes
- Bread
- Pasta mixes
- Sauce mixes
- Deep fried foods
- Frozen breakfast foods
- Packaged snacks
- Many different types of candies
- Some salted peanuts
- White bread
- Non-dairy creamers
- Tortillas
- Donuts
- Peanut butter
- Ice cream and low fat ice cream
- Hamburger and hot dog buns
- Movie popcorn
- Frozen pizza
- Refrigerated dough products

- Most fried foods—ask what type of oil the product is fried in
- Piecrust
- Cake mixes
- Pancakes and pancake mixes
- Waffles
- Frozen burgers
- Beef hot dogs
- Refrigerated cookie dough
- Biscuits and sweet rolls
- Refrigerated dough
- Breakfast sandwiches
- Meat sticks
- Crunchy noodles
- Canned chili
- Packaged pudding
- Fish sticks
- Low-fat ice cream
- Frozen burritos
- Noodle soup cups
- Cocoa or hot chocolate mix
- Instant mashed potatoes
- Gravy mixes
- Dips
- Potato chips
- Frozen pot pies
- Sandwiches grilled at a restaurant
- Reduced fat and fat free noodles
- Spreads

• Consider Eliminating Alcohol

At this time, it is best to stop all alcohol. A glass of wine occasionally when trying to get pregnant might not hurt, but nothing more and no hard liquors. Many studies suggest that the higher your alcohol consumption, the less chance you have of conceiving. Alcohol can impair the detoxifying process that occurs within the liver, and if the liver is working hard to metabolize alcohol, it can become run down and sick. Too much alcohol can also contribute to hormonal imbalances.

Alcohol can adversely affect ovulation and affect the body's ability to produce the amino acids necessary for cell development.

• Cut Down On White Flour Products

How many white flour products do you eat each day? Do you start your day with a bagel, donut or white bread toast? If so, get rid of white flour in your life as much as possible. An occasional bowl of spaghetti may be okay, but in general, you want to reduce the white flour products in your life as much as you can. White flour products, including pasta, bagels and bread, are not health builders and will not advance your goal of becoming pregnant. If you feel extremely weak and lethargic after eating white flour products, you may have celiac disease or a wheat intolerance. Symptoms include stomachaches, fatigue, bloating and flatulence. Check labels and brands. Some sources of white flour can include:

- Alcohol
- Crackers
- Cereals
- Corn flour
- Cake and cookie mixes
- Pancake mixes
- Muffin mixes
- Puddings
- Pretzels
- Donuts
- Foods with artificial colorings and preservatives
- Sweet and sour glazes
- Sweet sauces
- Soy sauce
- Ice cream cones
- Foods containing malt
- Powdered or canned soups
- Fast foods
- Gravies

Instead, choose wheat-free products made from rice, oat, rye, and puffed rice cereals.

• Reduce Your Intake Of Diet Foods or Foods with Sugar Substitutes

You may want to consider reducing your intake of diet foods, diet drinks or foods with sugar substitutes or artificial sweeteners. Some experts on fertility recommend avoiding sweeteners listed on labels as aspartame, sucralose, acesulfame potassium, also listed as acesulfame k and ACE, neotame, and saccharin.

Consider cutting back or eliminating diet drinks and powdered drinks that contain any of these sweeteners. These sweeteners may also be in some chewing gums and ice creams.

Some doctors have concluded that these artificial sweeteners interfere with fetal development, and act as 'instant birth control.' Aspartame is considered a endocrine disrupting chemical, by some medical providers.

Artificial sweeteners and sugar substitutes negatively impact the hormones in the pituitary glands, thyroid and ovaries.

Hidden sources of these artificial sweeteners can include:

• Breads
• Jello
• Gelatins
• Toothpaste
• Breath mints
• Drink mixes
• Syrups
• Jellies
• Cereals
• Sugar-free candies

• Reduce or Eliminate Soy

Some studies suggest that high levels of soy act as endocrine disrupters and decrease fertility. The phytoestrogens found in soy interfere with endocrine function and can mimic the female hormone oestrogen, which disrupts the normal production of sex hormones. Soy can decrease the follicle-stimulating hormone (FSH), as well as the leutinizing hormone.

Many soy products are genetically engineered and can reduce the body's ability to absorb minerals. Some soy isoflavones mimic estrogen—which means the body thinks it has estrogen it doesn't have, thus causing hormone imbalances. Some studies have also shown that soy can lead to thyroid problems, such as hypothyroidism.

Soy derivatives are often labeled under different names, including mono-diglyceride, soya, soja, yuba, TSF or textured soy flour, TSP textured soy protein, TVP textured vegetable protein, lecithin, and MSG, yeast extract, soy protein.

Hidden sources of soy include:

• Protein bars
• Meal replacement shakes
• Bottled fruit drinks
• Soups
• Sauces
• Baked goods
• Breakfast cereals
• Chewing gum
• Chocolate
• Bread
• Microwave meals
• Frozen pizzas
• Processed meat
• Soy milk
• Soy beans
• Corn chips
• Canned tuna

For more information on Fertility-Strengthening Foods, the entire version of Dancing Your Way to Fertility is available on www.amazon.com.

Your Personal Fertility Food Diary

It is important that every day, you keep track of what you eat. How healthy you become is closely related to the foods you take into your body.

There is a direct correlation between your level of fertility, vitality and energy and the foods and liquids you consume.

Ask yourself:

What foods make me feel stronger, brighten my mood, and give me energy?

What foods give me a second wind?

What foods leave me feeling exhausted?

What foods make me tired and cranky?

What live foods do I eat daily?

Breakfast: Say goodbye to cereal and milk, a bagel and coffee, pancakes and maple syrup. Say hello to oatmeal, blueberries and spinach.

Starting your diet with a few teaspoons of cooked spinach, maybe with a pinch or two of romano grated cheese. Other great breakfast choices: lots of walnuts, avocados and blueberries, a big bowl or romaine lettuce doused with olive oil. A big glass of juiced spinach and kale. A smoothie with spinach, maca, flax seed, blueberries and honey.

You have to replace all the ideas you've had about traditional breakfast foods, and replace them with foods that are alive, not laden down with corn syrup, sugar and white flour. The standard breakfast foods most of us eat can wreak havoc with our fertility. The goal each morning should be to eat nuts, beans, vegetables. No more lattes, coffees, or anything else caffeinated, white-floured or sugared to kick-start your day.

Lunch: Say goodbye to fast food lunches, deli meat, or lots of poor quality red meat.

Say hello to salads with things like walnuts and chick peas in them. Say goodbye to caffeine and soda to get through the day. No more chips with that tuna fish sandwich. A healthy lunch could include a salad with some chicken in it, homemade vegetable soup, with an apple, a grilled cheese with whole grain bread. A healthy lunch could also include a pumpkin-sunflower seed combination, or slices of pineapple drizzled with honey. A pita pocket filled with parsley, basil and kale, drizzled with olive oil and flaxseed oil.

Snacks: Snacks should include lots of healthy fruits, seeds, nuts, and vegetables. Candy bars, diet drinks or desserts, sugary desserts, chips, all should be eliminated.

Dinner: No white flour, trans fats, fast food, foods that contain msg or trans fats. Think lean proteins, healthy fish, lots of greens, salad, vegetables, nuts, and olive oil.

Your Personal Fertility Food Diary

Green Foods Eaten Today:

Fruits Eaten Today:

Vegetables Eaten Today:

Nuts Eaten Today:

Seeds Eaten Today:

Healthy Oils Eaten Today:

Vegetable and/or Fruit Drinks Made Today:

Diary Excerpt: Adjusting To A New Way of Life

 In many ways, starting infertility treatments is like starting a new life—one I wasn't exactly ready for. I tip toed into this process, rather than diving headfirst into it. When I first began, I didn't think a lot about what was happening—all I knew is I wanted a baby and I felt safe that I was in the hands of a reputable fertility clinic. I didn't analyze much or have a well thought-out strategy.

I suppose, looking back, my tip toe approach worked for me, but it was not one I had the luxury of staying with for very long.

I was not prepared for how demanding treatments can be...blood tests at 6 a.m., ultrasounds, more blood tests, shots every night. I was often late for my appointments. I had a hard time juggling my work schedule and the demands of the clinic. I had not yet altered my life enough to include fertility. It felt like an interruption I wasn't yet ready to surrender to.

I felt like the clinic was constantly calling me wanting something...another blood test, one more ultra-sound—didn't they realize that if went to the 6:30 a.m. ultrasound, I would be exhausted by the time I got out of work at 9 o'clock?

Surrender...that is the word that describes the process in many ways. Battling infertility takes battling, but it also takes surrender. For someone like me, I had to progress to the point where the requirements of the clinic had to take priority over my own exhaustion, work schedule, social life, or personal desires.

At a certain point, the only personal desire I had to pay attention to was my desire for a baby.

For the first six months, I was consistently late for most of my appointments. I sometimes didn't show up due to my work schedule or car problems. I did this so many times, I finally got called on the carpet by Dr. P.

"Are you ready for this?" he asked. He told me that if I continued to miss appointments or show up late, the clinic could not continue treating me.

Talk about a wake-up call.

Suddenly, I realized that I had to take this whole process very seriously and live up to whatever it was the clinic asked of me, even when it was hard. I could blow my opportunity to have what I most wanted due to my own irresponsible behavior.

I explained to Dr. P some of the problems caused by my work schedule, and a few car problems that caused me to miss appointments.

He understood, but made it clear that this type of behavior couldn't continue and was not acceptable.

If I wanted their help, I had to be responsible. If I wanted these treatments to work, I had to commit to doing whatever they asked. Whenever they wanted me there, I had to be there.

Looking back, I consider this the first step in my training for motherhood: being responsible isn't an option.

I walked out of that appointment somber and scared.

I wanted a baby, and I would have to put aside whatever was preventing me from getting to my appointments on time.

This was one of the many turning points in my treatment.

Dr. P was forcing me to make a choice: continue life as you know it, without 6 a.m. blood tests, or go through this painful, inconvenient, life-interrupting process in order to get what you want most.

I left knowing I had to change, and this was one of the many times my infertility treatments would push me in ways that I needed to be pushed in order to become the mother I wanted to be.

The Infertility Diaries can be purchased at www.amazon.com.

Chapter 2

Getting Your Guy Ready: The Ultimate Male Fertility Preparation Program

Along with getting yourself prepared for pregnancy, it is important to help your husband and/or partner become as fertile as possible. Don't panic if your guy was diagnosed with a low sperm count. Just as there are many things a woman can do to maximize her fertility, there are also many things a man can do to improve the quality, quantity, and speed of his sperm.

Whether or not your guy was diagnosed with any specific problem, it is important to address his fertility because underlying, undiagnosed problems could exist that are not being caught.

Some causes of inadequate sperm production include hormone imbalances, post-testicular issues with plumping or ejaculation, trauma or accidents, varicocele, or dilated veins in the scrotum, undescended testis/testes, excessive xenoestrogen, which are environmental estrogen exposure; infectious disease of the epidydimis, a diseased endocrine (glandular) system affecting the hypothalamus, pituitary, thyroid, adrenals and the testes, resulting in low DHEA and testosterone levels, congenital abnormalities, urethral stricture, malnutrition, especially protein deficiency.

It can sometimes take two to three months to improve the quality of sperm, so you'll want to begin preparing as soon as possible.

Tests For Men

Here are some of the tests your husband/partner can request:

• Sperm analysis, including a sperm antibody test, which can determine sperm count, motility, morphology (shape), seminal fluid, volume of ejaculation, and pH level.

• A Hormone Analysis: Hormones include testosterone, follicle stimulating hormone, and lutinizeing hormone which are critical to sperm production. You may also want to have analyzed prolacin levels, thyroid stimulating hormone, sand ex-hormone binding globulin.

• Scrotal Doppler Ultrasound: measures the size of the testicle and look for blockages that involve transport of sperm out of the testicle.

• Transrectal Ultrasound: ultrasound technology is used to image the reproductive tract.

• A blood test to check for infections and hormone levels.

• A white blood cell count to detect infection, past infection, inflammation, low levels of inhibin B, or the compound alpha-glucosidase.

• Forward progression: this test measures the amount of forward movement in the sperm.

• Kruger morphology: if an abnormal morphology is found, this test allows the specialists to examine the sperm structure in great detail.

• Anti-sperm antibodies: this means the male has created an immunological response toward the sperm cells

• Sperm agglutination: sperm is examined to see whether there is any clumping together of the cells. Sperm agglutination can indicate the presence of sperm antibodies or bacterial infection.

• Viability: this test is performed if the sperm analysis shows that less than 30 percent of the sperm are motile. This test determines whether or not there is a presence of live sperm.

• Fructose: this test determines whether there is a blockage or no sperm at all being produced.

• An often overlooked cause of infertility in men is low-grade infection in the male urinary tract. Symptoms are often subtle and hard to diagnose, but they can include chills, fever, increased urination and intense burning during urination. Some physicians recommend culturing a semen sample to detect this mild infection.

• Cleanses

Here are some cleanses for men to consider before beginning infertility treatments.

• **A Parasite Cleanse:** Parasites can weaken sperm on a very hard-to-detect level. Health food stores carry 30-day parasite cleanses that can effectively remove parasites from the body.

• **Heavy Metal Cleanse:** Chemicals, pesticides and toxins in our environment have greatly impacted male fertility. Many men suffer from low-quality sperm because of these environmental toxins and chemicals. If possible, consider a heavy metal cleanse that can help remove these chemicals.

• **Liver Cleanse:** Just as detoxifying the liver is key to healing female infertility, it is equally important for men. Consider having your partner do a liver cleanse. The liver helps to filter toxins from the body, including excess hormones.

• **Candida-Yeast Cleanse:** can help rid the body of toxins.

• **Colon Hydrotherapy:** A colon cleanse can eradicate years of toxins in the large intestine, reducing the burden on the liver, pancreas, gall bladder and kidney.

• Holistic and Alternative Health Treatments to Consider

• **Acupuncture:** Acupuncture has been known to help men who have a low sperm count. It may be helpful for your partner to begin weekly or twice-weekly acupuncture treatments.
Make sure to let the acupuncturist know that you are looking to strengthen your husband's sperm Acupuncture points can help redirect Qi (energy) to key points in the body that assist in the smooth flow of blood to the penis and scrotum.

• Vitamins and Supplements

Here are some vitamins and supplements that can often help male infertility:

• **Vitamin C:** High-quality vitamin C supplements enhance sperm development. Some recommend 2,000 to 6,000 milligrams daily to prevent sperm from clumping or sticking together.

Foods that contain lots of Vitamin C include strawberries, citrus fruits, cherries, cantaloupe, broccoli, tomatoes, sweet peppers, mangos, kiwi, pineapple, grapes, peas, potatoes, parsley and spinach. Keep a bowl of these foods washed and easily available.

• **Zinc:** is very important to sperm quality because it increases testosterone levels, sperm count and sperm motility. Men should consider taking a zinc supplement or a high-quality multivitamin that contains zinc, as a zinc deficiency has been shown to cause or reduce male infertility.

In addition to taking a supplement, foods high in zinc include oysters, organic meats, lean beef, turkey, lamb, herring, wheat germ, beans, sunflower and pumpkin seeds.

• **L-Arginine:** is an amino acid that enhances low sperm counts and poor motility. It is found in high amounts in the head of the sperm. Studies show that sperm and semen volume double with this amino acid.

Food sources of L-arginine include nuts, raisins, sesame seeds, brown rice, peanuts, almonds chocolate, meat and poultry.

• **A Multivitamin:** taken daily.

• **Vitamin E:** Studies have shown that Vitamin E increases sperm health and motility.

• **Folic acid:** Studies suggest that men with low levels of this key B vitamin have trouble producing healthy sperm. Folic acid reportedly improves sperm motility and sperm structure. Food sources include leafy greens, orange juice and spinach.

• **Korean Ginseng:** enhances testosterone and sperm levels.

• **Selenium:** should be taken as part of a quality multi-vitamin.

• **Coenzyme Q10:** increases energy production in the sperm and can increase motility and quality of sperm.

• **Omega-3:** acts as a hormone regulator.

• **Vitamin A:** helps enhance male hormones.

• **B-complex:** This vitamin is very important to male fertility. Vitamin B6 and B12 have been reported to improve sperm counts. Vitamin B12 can increase the quantity and quality of your guy's sperm. Foods that contain B vitamins include lamb, sardines and salmon.

• **Calcium-Magnesium:** aids Vitamin B absorption.

• **Vitamin A:** increases male hormones. Eat plenty of vegetables, fruit, oily fish and dark green leafy vegetables.

• **Royal Jelly:** can help optimize hormonal balance.

• **Manganese deficiency:** is known to result in testicular degeneration. Foods with manganese include: whole grains, green vegetables, carrots, broccoli, beans, nuts, pineapples, oats, rye and eggs.

• Things Your Guy Can Do To Improve His Fertility

• **Visit The Dentist:** Make sure your husband has his teeth cleaned, thus eliminating the possibility of infections in the gums or teeth.

• **Consider His Weight:** Too much or too little body fat can disrupt production of reproductive hormones, thus reducing sperm count. Try to help your husband/partner lose weight, especially scrotal fat, which can act like a warm blanket over the scrotum and elevate sperm temperatures, which in turn, kill and immobilize sperm. Excess fat around the waist is often associated with decreased male fertility.

• **Reduce Stress:** Encourage your husband/partner to take steps to reduce stress, as stress has been shown to negatively impact male reproductive hormones and lower testosterone.

• **Drink Lots of Water:** Make sure your partner is drinking plenty of high-quality, filtered water each day.

• **Touch, Touch and Touch Some More:** Stimulation increases hormones and improves fertility. Touch each other at length before intercourse to increase hormones, both his and yours.

• **Ejaculate Often:** Sex is good for sperm, because the less time spent in storage, the higher quality it will be and less DNA damage.

• **Enjoy More Sunshine:** Encourage your guy to get outside 10 to 15 minutes a day.

• **Alkalize His Body With Greens:** Lots of healthy vegetables can help restore the acid-alkaline balance in the reproductive system to the proper sperm pH. A diet high in acid-producing foods such as meat, white flour, sugar, alcohol, coffee and soft drinks is to be avoided.

For more on Getting Your Guy Ready and the Ultimate Male Fertility Preparation Program, including what your guy should avoid to protect his fertility and fertility enhancing foods for men, Dancing Your Way to Fertility can be purchased at www.amazon.com.

Chapter 3: How To Prepare For the Journey Through Infertility

• Prepare To Take Responsibility for Your Own Healing

This journey is your responsibility and yours alone. Your journey to motherhood is not the responsibility of your doctor, your husband, your mother, or your best friend.

You will ultimately fare better if you take responsibility for your infertility treatments, rather than hoping someone is going to come and pave the way for you or rescue you.

You are in charge and responsible for all the hard work your infertility treatments will demand and require.

Accepting the responsibility of finding a good doctor, showing up to all your appointments, and doing whatever it takes to heal your body, will empower you to make good choices, be organized, self-disciplined, and do whatever you can to improve your chances of conceiving the baby you so deserve.

You are the one that must go to the appointments, take the medications, change whatever needs to be changed and sacrifice whatever needs to be sacrificed, in the quest to have a baby. You are in charge. You make the choices. You ask the questions. You do the research. You explore your options. You ask to try another medication. You change doctors. You eat healthy. You show up on time for the appointments. The choices, the actions, are all up to you.

You want this baby, you need to understand you are the driver. You are not a child resting easily in the arms of your doctor or anyone else.

Relying on the word of any one doctor, or any one clinic, or any one person, is a big mistake. Starting right now, you need to take responsibility for your treatment--not hand it over to anyone or rely totally on anyone else.

Many women have made the mistake of letting the course of their treatment be dictated by one person--usually a medical professional--only to find out later that person had been on the wrong track.

By putting yourself firmly in the driver's seat, you will not be afraid to ask for things, push for more, change course when you see the need. You will not be tethered to a treatment that is not working for you. Nor will you be a victim to whatever some authority figure sees fit for you, especially if their pronouncement or decision isn't bringing you the desired results.

Stay in charge and realize that no one can run this race for you but you.

Taking responsibility does not mean blaming yourself, hating yourself, or beating yourself when you hit hard times and disappointments. It is not your fault when a cycle doesn't work out and you are not pregnant yet. Taking responsibility means educating yourself, speaking up for yourself, advocating for yourself, believing in yourself. You need to understand and fully realize that you--and only you--are responsible and in charge of your infertility treatments and journey.

• Prepare To Talk Positively To Yourself Each Day

Starting now, you need to tell yourself every single day that your body can and will get pregnant and give birth.

Say right out loud that your body is healing from infertility, that it is only a temporary condition, and that you are capable, able and strong enough to have a baby.

Repeat over and over again that your body is ready, willing and able to receive and nurture a new life.

It is key that right from the start of this journey, you understand the importance of your self-talk. At this time, you must be your own best friend, your personal cheerleader, your own fertility coach, as you consciously choose to speak words of hope, health and healing to your body.

What you speak aloud and what you speak internally must be positive. No dire pronouncements. No words like, "I'll never get pregnant" or "this won't work out."

You must commit right now that you will speak to your body in a way that
encourages healing, confidence, success, and growth.

All the self-hating, blaming words must end now.

Stop the negative self-talk that the body listens to, and ultimately obeys, on an unconscious level.

Start talking to yourself and your body, both silently and aloud, about the success and healing you are soon going to experience. You need to tell your body that yes, you are going to have a baby. Yes, you are going to be a parent. Your self-talk needs to be affirm a good and beautiful outcome for your efforts.

Let your body know you love it and you have faith it will find a way to conceive, carry and give birth to a beautiful baby.

Let your ovaries, vagina, kidneys, adrenal glands and liver know that you love them and you believe in their power. Hug yourself, soothe yourself. Stop the voices in your head that call you weak, powerless, sickly, infertile.

Never ever say "this won't work."

When you are feeling down and you can sense that your internal whisperings are going to be negative, stop and envision how lovingly you would talk to a friend in this situation.

Just as you need to talk kindly to yourself, be aware of the words you use when speaking to others about your infertility. Even if you feel discouraged, NEVER EVER say out loud, "I doubt I will get pregnant" or "I don't think this will happen for me."
Repeat: even during difficult times, never let negative words that predict an unhappy outcome for your efforts escape from your lips.

• Prepare to Say Goodbye to Guilt, Shame and Self-Blame

Infertility is not a weakness, a curse, or a sin. Infertility is not something you should feel guilty about.

It is not your fault and it certainly doesn't mean you are not meant to be a mother.

Infertility is a temporary physical condition that can be treated and healed. Millions of women once diagnosed with infertility went on to heal and give birth to their babies.

Should a person with a bad cold feel guilty because their nose is running? Doesn't a person with a cold take Vitamin C and rest, knowing that with some orange juice and chicken soup, their nose will eventually stop running and they will return to living without a cold?

Is a person with cancer somehow to blame for the cancer? No, the body sometimes gets on the wrong track, and whether it is a runny nose, an arthritic knee, cancer or acne, we should never blame ourselves for the times when the body goes awry. We are not physically perfect, nor should we expect ourselves to be.

What we are, and what we can expect from ourselves, is the capacity to heal and renew from temporary physical conditions.

Instead of guilt and shame, we need to forgive our body, love our body, be kind and good to our body, and work slowly and lovingly towards healing our body. Illness is in no way a reason to engage in self-hatred.

The body cannot be beaten and shamed back into health. It can, however, be loved and soothed back to a healthy state.

Wipe away right now any archaic ideas that you are evil, flawed, or cursed because you are having trouble getting pregnant.

You are not a bad person because you have a physical problem with conception.

You are in simply a temporary state of infertility that can be healed.

Infertility is a malfunction of the body, just like any illness, and it is no reason to beat yourself up.
Does infertility make you less of a woman? No, no and no. No self-hate allowed. No needless shame or guilt is warranted. You need now to love yourself as much as possible.

What is there to be ashamed of? What is there to feel guilty about?

Infertility is not a statement about your character, your worth, your power as a woman, your ability to mother, your maternal calling, your right to be a mother, your childhood, your family history, your ability to mother, or anything else. Infertility is the result of the body straying down an unhealthy track—a track, however, that you can lovingly lead your body away from so that you can ultimately get back on a healthy, vibrant, blooming and yes, fertile track.

Say a goodbye to emotions like guilt and self-hatred because there is no validity to them.

• Prepare As If You Were A Professional Runner Training For A Race

While going through infertility, consider yourself a runner training for a race. Professional runners are aware that there are many obstacles that can come up during a race and they prepare ahead of time for them.

Successful runners develop the trait of resilience, which gives them the power to bounce back from setbacks. They acknowledge the setback, but quickly move past it so they can focus on the goal ahead.

They know the importance of developing mental toughness and strength so they can continue running, regardless of the conditions, distractions, and emotions they experience during a race.

A successful runner develops the ability to keep moving forward towards their goal, even when there are no immediate signs of winning or even being closer to the finish line. They develop an inner voice that says, 'I can do this. I have the resources inside of me to succeed.' They keep running towards their goal, even when the finish line seems impossible to reach. Some runners write positive sayings on their arms or water bottles so they have a motivational thought to carry them through. Some runners keep themselves going by visualizing how it will feel to get to the finish line and win the race.

While going through your infertility treatments, you plan ahead and prepare a strategy to follow even during the rough times. You develop a mental toughness, so you can bounce back from disappointment, whether or not anyone is cheering you on or believes you can win.

You follow your plan of action, even when your goal seems elusive or faraway. You keep listening to that positive inner voice that says: 'yes, you can get pregnant' even when the finish line is nowhere in sight.

• Prepare To Connect To Your Body

Stop hating your curves, dreading your 'time of the month' and disliking the shape and size of your breasts. No, they are NOT too big/too small/too whatever. They are just perfect.

Stop hating the smells that come from your vagina or underarms.

Stop. Just stop.

Its time to start embracing your womanly, feminine body.

This includes your menstrual cycle, your pubic hair, your shapely (or not so shapely) backside.

Start honoring your period. No bad mouthing it, please. It is part of the birth cycle. Stop denying it and suppressing it. Love it and appreciate it.

Your body, in all its amazing womanliness, is trying to do its best for you. Say thank you to it. Give it a big hug. Show some gratitude.

For more on how to prepare for the journey through infertility, the entire version of Dancing Your Way to Fertility can be purchased at www.amazon.com.

Chapter 4: Emotions That Can Come From Suffering With Infertility

There are very difficult emotions that being an infertility patient will bring up within you.

Yes, you have every right to feel rage, jealousy, anger, resentment, fear and intense sadness. Infertility is hell. Pure and simple.

You have been through a lot.

You have a right to have a baby, and none of this is fair.

Having your life plan delayed can be frustrating and maddening.

It is not fair in any way that you should have to wait so long and suffer so much for something that is your natural birthright.

Being a mother may be something you drept of and wanted since you were a little girl. When it doesn't happen the way you once thought it would happen, you can feel devastated. Completely alone. Cast away on an island you never wanted to. Isolated from the life you imagined you would have.

Then, there are the daily injections, early morning ultrasounds, and month-to-month cycles that don't always work out, that can leave you angry, emotionally exhausted, grief-stricken and jealous.

Sometimes, you don't want to talk about it. You definitely don't want to be lectured about it. And you certainly don't want to hear one more stupid, insensitive person make a comment like 'just relax and it will happen.'

So you stay silent. Friends and family have no idea of the dark pit infertility patients sometimes end up in.

Going to social events can be painful, especially when they center around celebrations involving pregnancy, birth and children.

Here are a few ways to cope with some of the feelings and emotions that accompany infertility treatments:

Anger: Infertility is hell (I said it before and I will say it again) and if you feel angry about the whole thing, you have every right to feel that way. We feel angry when we are frustrated and unable to get what we want.

Anger is an emotion that is often a combination of feeling powerless, afraid and hurt.

Anger sometimes appears in the form of resentment, irritability, rage, animosity, and bitterness.

In Chinese medicine it is believed that anger affects the liver, which is a key organ in infertility. The more you release the toxins in your liver, the less your body will be able to hold onto anger.

There are also alternative/holistic therapies that can help release anger, such as craniosacral/myofascial therapy, acupuncture, and homeopathy. Massage and trauma release can also help release anger. Swimming can be a safe way to release anger. I started swimming when I began infertility treatments, and once found myself sobbing after a very intense swim. I didn't know why I was crying, but I sensed my body was releasing pent-up anger.

Spending time in nature, sitting by the ocean, are also ways to release anger.

When you begin to feel anger, try to do one thing that gives you a feeling of control in your life, such as juicing a green drink, saying a positive affirmation, or going to an acupuncture appointment. Close your eyes and picture the part of you that is angry and ask that part of you: what can I give you right now that will help you feel better?

Let your inner child know you will help her have the baby she so desires. Comfort her. Ask her: what is it you want honey? Then listen closely for the answers.

Remember: anger is a secondary emotion. There is something you feel before you feel angry. Try to identify what emotions you feel before you reach anger.

When you begin to feel angry, say: 'I am powerful. I am powerful and able to get what I want.'

Do something creative that gives your anger a chance leave your body and take another form outside of yourself.

Anger does not have to trap you into a helpless state that leaves your body stressed. Acknowledge it, give yourself something that it needs, and release it when you can.

Jealousy: Jealousy is an emotion everyone feels at one time or another, regardless of our circumstances and situations in life. We all feel jealous when we see someone with something we desperately want, but don't have. It is easy to feel jealous of women who have children. Don't feel guilty about experiencing this emotion. Jealousy often comes from a perceived scarcity in an area of your life. So rather than seeing other people's babies as a slap in the face, begin to see it as a cue that 'if it is possible for them, it is possible for me.'

The next time you see a mother with her children and you feel jealous, say to yourself: if it could happen to her, it could happen to me.

Think of it this way: her success today mirrors the potential for your success tomorrow.

When you hear of a baby shower or find out a friend is pregnant, it means that pregnancy and birth are conditions possible in our world— possible for them and possible for you.

Realize that just because you don't have something today doesn't mean you won't have it tomorrow.

Try, (I know how hard this is) to keep a vision of a tomorrow where you have the babies you deserve.

Repeat: 'There is enough to go around.' 'There is enough for everybody.' 'I too can have what I want.' 'I will have a baby too.'

When you see a baby, repeat the words: 'babies are born, babies are here, babies are everywhere, and my baby is coming too.' Or: 'this just proves that babies are always coming and my baby is coming too.'

Feeling robbed and jealous are not emotions that just disappear overnight. Nor should you feel guilty when you experience them. Just keep reminding yourself that every baby you see is a reminder that babies are born everyday—and one of these days it could very well be your baby that is born! Keep a note on your refrigerator that says: "There is enough for everybody! There is enough for me! Lots of women have babies and I will have one too!"

For more on the emotions that can come from suffering with infertility, such as frustration, grief and jealousy, visit www.amazon.com to purchase Dancing Your Way to Fertility.

Chapter 5: Coping With The Ups and Downs of Infertility Treatments

How do you not go crazy when you run into an old friend who has three beautiful kids and just announced she is happily pregnant with her fourth?

How do you keep going, when the shots, the appointments, the painful tests, seem never ending?

How do you persevere when the nurse calls again with another, 'no, I'm sorry' message.

Sometimes, not being able to get pregnant is nothing short of torture, anguish, a raw clawing frustration, because what is natural is not coming naturally.

There were times during my infertility treatments when I was hysterical, depressed, unable to be consoled.

This is no easy time and no easy task.

There will be times when you will rightly feel very angry, frustrated and even downright hopeless. My guess is that you are a lot stronger than you think you are, but feelings are feelings and sometimes they are just there and can't be ignored.

Here's what five years of infertility treatments taught me about coping with the ups and downs that accompany this difficult and trying process.

• Accept That Some Days You Are Just Going To Fall Apart

There are going to be days when it all gets too much. The unfairness of what you are going through, the longing for a child that continues to be unfulfilled, the raw pain of seeing a world filled with pregnant women and babies, and you somehow denied that joy, will all get too much. When that happens, you might collapse into bed, cry uncontrollably, rage at your husband, flip out at the next friend who tells you to just relax. You won't always behave appropriately, you might do unproductive things. Sometimes you might just feel like the pain of it all is going to kill you.

Knowing ahead of time that this might happen won't relieve you of the pain, but it might help you remember that thousands of women who experienced infertility also have had bad days like this—and thousands of them now have children. Eventually, many of them got pregnant and gave birth, despite heartbreaking disappointments.
That lady you walked by in the supermarket with the adorable kids who made your heart ache? She very well could have been an infertility patient once upon a time.

Know this: you may be crying hysterically today because you are not pregnant, and a year or two from now, you might be spending your day taking care of your sweet baby.

• In Your Darkest Moments, Remember What Choices Are Still Available to You

During the moments when you feel you can't take anymore, ask yourself this question: what is one thing I can do today that will move me one step closer to my goal?

You got a call and the news was bad: no, you are not pregnant. In that moment of complete disappointment, stop and ask yourself: what is one positive action I can do right now to help me get one step closer to having a baby? Before you fall apart, before you start crying, ask yourself this one question and immediately take a step towards this positive action.

• Take Control Of What You Can Control

 To cope with all the things that happen during infertility that are out of your control, learn to take control of what you can control. You have control over what enters your mouth and what you put on our skin. You have control over what type of water you drink, what types of cleaning chemicals you use in your home and yard, and what types of holistic healing you bring into your life. During your moments of despair, grab hold of what is still under your control and do the best, most positive, healing action available to you. What you can control, control well.

• Keep the 'Happy Chemicals' In Your Brain Flowing

 Work hard to make sure the 'happy' chemicals in your brain are working at their maximum capacity. Infertility can be devastating to your emotional self, so try to counteract it by revving up the happy-chemicals your brain. Exercise gently, eat lots of green vegetables, get lots of sleep, reduce your coffee intake and take extra folic acid.

Research has shown that embracing a positive new goal stimulates the release of dopamine, believing in yourself triggers serotonin. Putting yourself around people you trust releases oxytocin. Sniffing vanilla and lavender releases endorphins. Knitting or sewing can give you feelings similar to meditation. To enhance your positive experiences, write them down.

For more information on coping with the ups and downs of infertility, the entire version of Dancing Your Way to Fertility can be purchased at www.amazon.com.

Chapter 6: The People In Your Journey and Some of the Rude Comments You May Hear Along the Way

This is not to be misinterpreted as an exercise in dumping family or friends, because people are not perfect and we should not expect them to be, and there are people in our lives, as unpleasant as they may be, that we simply need to forgive, stay connected to and be around. Despite their flaws, we owe them something. That being said, as you walk this journey, you need to be ready for some of the stupid, rude and totally insensitive comments you are going to hear. Sometimes, people you love will say really dumb things. Other times, it could be a stranger who zaps you with a statement that leaves you breathless and feeling punched in the gut.

Here are a few of the stupid, rude, thoughtless and COMPLETELY FALSE comments you may have to deal with, and how best to respond:

• **"Maybe you weren't meant to have a baby":** Yes, you were meant to have a baby. Yes, you were. Millions of women have babies whether they want them or not, whether they will be good mothers or not, so why shouldn't you have a baby? In fact, there is NOT ONE REASON IN THIS UNIVERSE why you should not have a baby.

This person is either jealous of you or just likes to pop the balloon of hope. People who mouth off a comment like this mistakenly feel they have some sort of moral authority. Ignore them. They are wrong. Completely and utterly wrong.

• "Aren't you a little too old to be trying for a baby?"

Whoever got the idea that a young mother is better than an older mother has not seen the millions of mothers in their 40s and even 50s who mother with great patience, love, insight, wisdom and kindness.

This person obviously doesn't understand that with age comes maturity and wisdom.

Someone who makes a comment like this may be focusing on the energy level of children, forgetting that even most 25 year old mothers are not out playing baseball with their kids everyday.

Whoever throws out a comment about age is ignorant of the fact that a woman of any age who is ready and able to love a child, and who is brave and strong enough to endure infertility, is more prepared, capable and ready to mother than almost anyone.

A good mother is a good mother, whether she is 21, 31, 41, 51 or beyond.

For more on the rude comments you may hear along the way, visit www.amazon.com to purchase a copy of Dancing Your Way to Fertility.

Chapter 7: A Note About Husbands and How To Not Let Infertility Ruin Your Marriage

Here are my thoughts about husbands:

Infertility can be rough on a marriage.

From the day you start infertility treatments, it will be best if you let go of the idea that your husband will always be able to fully understand and care for all the emotions you will experience in the quest to have a baby.

Let go of the idea that he will always say the right thing. Abandon the hope that he will always know exactly how to comfort you.

As much as my husband wanted children, he did not always understand my raw anguish or single-minded drive. Looking back, I shouldn't have expected him to understand all my emotions. It was a waste of time and energy I needed to put into my healing.

What I didn't understand was that, while my husband's desire to have children was strong, he manifested it differently than I did.

Sometimes I became enraged when I felt he was being a bit too clinical about the whole experience.

Don't try to get your husband to express his desire for a baby in the exact same way you do. It is pointless. Your husband cannot be the focus of your frustration right now.

Doing things to make your body healthier is where your energy needs to be, not in fighting with your husband over his perceived insensitivities.

Some husbands are just not able to fully grasp the intense passion, fervor and sometimes obsession a woman can feel over having a baby.

If your husband does understand, you are very fortunate.

If not, that's okay too.

Just remember--this journey isn't about him--it is about bringing the baby of your dreams to life. Wasting time arguing with him or expecting him to totally relate to your feelings is, well, a waste of time.

As much as you need his support right now, you need to empower yourself and find your strength within. If you can, build a network of support outside of your marriage, so that he won't be your exclusive source of comfort.

Don't expect him to rescue you from the pain and work involved in infertility treatments. Don't expect him to mother you, nurse you, or completely get what this means to you.

Do expect he may say exactly what you don't want him to say at exactly the wrong time.

Many husbands end up becoming true heroes to their wives during infertility treatments, but even those who rise to the challenge can sometimes disappoint--not because they are insensitive or uncaring, but simply because they might be tired, cranky, or feeling intense emotions of their own.

Infertility is tiring and sometimes people run out of steam.

For the times when perhaps he is insensitive, forgive him and let it go. Don't waste time moping and groaning about how he doesn't get it.

Remember: your husband cannot save you from the pain of this ordeal, or erase the frustration and rage you sometimes are going to feel.

Don't make trying to get him to understand your feelings your mission-- you will be wasting precious time and emotional resources. Don't expect him to be driven in exactly the same way you are, although some men are.

For more on how to not let infertility ruin your marriage, an entire copy of Dancing Your Way to Fertility can be purchased at www.amazon.com.

Chapter 8: Choosing The Right Doctor

Don't underestimate the importance of having a good doctor, and don't ever be naive about the damage the wrong doctor can do. Frankly, the wrong doctor can steal your chance of having a baby and the family you dream of.

Start by researching infertility clinics in your area. You want to choose a clinic with high success rates and an esteemed reputation. You want a doctor who is a fertility specialist and affiliated with a highly reputable fertility clinic with a high success rate. I would strongly suggest against using your gynecologist as your infertility specialist.

A gynecologist may not have as much experience as a specialist who focuses exclusively on infertility. They may also lack the resources and access to the latest reproductive technologies.

Research the success rates of various clinics within 30 minutes to an hour from your home. When choosing a clinic, weigh carefully the travel time and route to the clinic. You will be going to the clinic a lot, sometimes every day for weeks. If travel is no consideration, go to the best clinic within an hour from you.

When choosing a clinic, make sure they have a wide range of fertility treatments available and are familiar with the latest technologies. If you have choices, try to select a clinic that makes you feel comfortable, doesn't stress you out, and who can offer you the best and most choices. If you know others dealing with infertility, ask for their opinions and experiences at different clinics with different doctors. I found the doctor who helped me become pregnant with my son through a neighbor he also helped conceive and give birth to her son.

It is important that you select a doctor you feel comfortable with and who answers your questions.

If a doctor refuses to answer your questions or seems to dismiss your questions, this may not be the doctor to select.

If they almost come off as disrespectful and arrogant, than perhaps then you need to ask yourself: will they listen if I request a certain test or change in medications? Or will they ignore my requests?

Ideally, you want a doctor who listens to your recommendations and orders whatever tests and medications you request.

A doctor who doesn't put the time into finding solutions for you may not be the right doctor.

While physicians in the infertility industry are very busy and it is not realistic to expect excessive emotional support, you should be able to expect one who listens and pays attention to your requests, is determined to help you, and is willing to try new procedures and medications. Some fertility doctors may seem cold because they have large caseloads.

Occasionally, doctors with high success rates can sometimes have a hidden agenda in trying to get you to quit the attempt for a biological child. Before following the recommendations of a doctor, always consider where their motive for your course of treatment might be coming from. If you are of an advanced age, every time you do an IUI or an IVF and it fails, their success rates for live births are lowered, and thus it is in their best interests to persuade you to try an alternative method that precludes the attempt at a biological child so their statistics remain high. Could your continuing to pursue the goal of having biological children lower their live birth rate statistics? Is this a doctor more concerned with their stats than with helping you achieve your goal? For those who can maintain high live birth statistics, it means higher rankings and more customers.

Also stay alert to how long you are kept on a medication, especially if it is not working. Is your doctor keeping track of your progress and alert to when a change in medication is needed? If you have suffered miscarriages, did your doctor prescribe or suggest progesterone for future pregnancies?

Are they making an attempt to give you what you need so you don't miscarry again?

Do not stay with a doctor who is not producing results for you, or at least trying to find what is going to work for you. If your doctor stays with the same protacol repeatedly, despite no success, it might be time to get another doctor. Or at least see if your doctor is willing to sit down and reevaluate your treatment plan.

For more information on choosing the right doctor, the entire version of Dancing Your Way to Fertility can be purchased at www.amazon.com.

Chapter 9: Common Mistakes You Need To Know About

Here are some common mistakes those suffering with infertility often encounter:

Waiting too long to get help: Stop listening to those people who tell you to simply relax and it will happen. Relaxing does help, but it is not the only solution. If you've been trying to get pregnant for awhile and it is not happening, see an infertility specialist immediately.

Not trying enough times and/or giving up too soon: When undergoing infertility treatments, never forget the old saying, "if at first you don't succeed, try, try again." Even if you have done several cycles, if you feel you can cope and want to continue, let yourself try again. Don't listen to those who say, 'you've tried X number of times and if it hasn't work yet it isn't going to.' The next try could be the one that works.

Not seeing the correlation between poor eating habits, and infertility: Don't get tricked into believing that you can eat any way you want and it won't impact your fertility. Everything you consume impacts your fertility—and it your responsibility to start getting this part of your life right.

Not strengthening every part of your body, from your liver, to your kidney to your adrenal glands: You know various ways to detoxify and strengthen your organs—so go ahead and do it.

Not participating in your own healing process and thinking it is someone else's responsibility: Your doctor and the infertility clinic can provide you with a treatment plan and medications to help you get pregnant, but the rest of the healing is up to you.

Not Trying To Discover The Root Cause of Your Infertility: Even if your doctor diagnoses you with 'unexplained infertility' the bottom line is there is a reason you are not getting pregnant—one that perhaps is so subtle that the clinics have no precise test that can diagnose it.

That is where it is in your best interests to seek out holistic and alternative medicine to address the subtle reasons your body is not conceiving naturally.

Chapter 10: Bye Bye Stress!

You've heard it a million times before. Now you will hear it again: stress is a huge enemy of your fertility. Stress weakens your body, impacts your hormones, and could be what is standing between you and your future children.

Stress makes your body a less welcoming and hospitable place. Some doctors believe that stress plays a role in 20 to 30 percent of all infertility cases.

The reason stress is so dangerous to your fertility is it elevates hormones like cortisol and epinephrine, which inhibit the body's main sex hormone gonadotropin releasing hormone (GnRH).

Stress inhibits the release of reproductive hormones. GnRH is responsible for the pituitary gland's release of luteinizing hormones and follicle-stimulating hormones.

Stress disrupts hormone communication between your brain, pituitary and ovaries, thus interfering with the maturation of the egg and ovulation process.

Stress can also kick the body into a fight or flight response that makes it difficult for the body to feel safe enough to get pregnant.

However, it should be noted that all around the world, lots of women are very stressed and get pregnant anyways. Stress is part of life, and yes, you will feel stressed sometimes during this process. I am not in any way saying: 'relax you will get pregnant' because there are many underlying, hard to detect physical reasons pregnancy is not occurring. It is disrespectful to suggest that a person going through infertility treatments would somehow not feel stressed.

Of course you are going to be stressed! How could you not? So, don't feel guilty if sometimes you feel stressed.

However, you deserve to stack the odds in your favor, and do whatever you can to reduce the stress hormones in your body.

Here are some suggestions:

• Take Some Time to Analyze Exactly What in Your Life Stresses You

For a few days, write down every time you feel stressed. What caused you to feel stressed? Where were you? Who were you with? What was happening that made you feel this way? Then, ask yourself: are these stressors something I can change?

Write down ways you can change the stress triggers in your life. If these stressors are not factors you can change, ask yourself: can I change my attitude or how I talk to myself about these stressors so I do not get as upset next time?

The goal is to identify your stressors and find ways to change your circumstances so these triggers are no longer in your life. Or, if you cannot change the stressful situations in your life, can you change the way you react, think, talk to yourself about, and cope with these stressors?

An example: you realize that your daily commute to work is very stressful. Is there an alternative route you could take? A co-worker you could drive in with? A form of public transportation that would be more relaxing? A favorite CD or book you could play while you drive to help change your mood and what you think about as you drive? Would your employer be open to a change in work schedule that might lessen the traffic you encounter?

Are there any opportunities for jobs closer to home or work-from-home days? What could you say to yourself during your commute that you can change? Start thinking of ways to address the situations that bring up feelings of stress in your life.

• Repeat Positive Sayings and Positive Words

If you find you get stressed around a certain person or at a certain time of day, choose a saying or mantra that you can repeat over and over to yourself that will help calm you down.

Sayings that might help include:

Let go and let God
With God all things are possible
Everything will be all right
Been there, done that, all will turn out well
Breathe, breathe, breathe
Time for my bath
This too shall pass
Keep calm and carry on
Keep calm and love
I don't worry, I be happy
I s-m-i-l-e
I don't have to be perfect
I choose happy
I choose good
The sun is shining on me
Right now, a batch of warm chocolate chips cookies are coming out of the oven
I breathe peace
I breathe love
Stay calm—it will be all right
Inch by inch, life's a cinch
One bite at a time
Relax, God is in charge
God loves me and will take care of me
Love is here right now
It will be okay
I did good
Peace is mine
I will conquer
I smile with joy
My happy heart is light

Love is here, love is mine, love is everywhere
Courage is mine
My heart is smiling
Hope arrived!
I stand by you
Life is beautiful
Once upon a time there was a princess named <u>your name here</u>
I am happy
I feel wonderful
I am love

Choose a mantra that elicits positive feelings within you. For example, if you relax when you hear the word 'chocolate' or 'joy' create a saying you can repeat each day around those words, such as 'I have chocolate covered joy."

• Put Yourself In Situations Or Around People That Make You Feel Safe

 Feelings of danger often bring up stress in the body. Do whatever you can to increase your feelings of safety at this time. If you feel safe wrapped in a certain blanket drinking tea, make that part of your daily routine. If hearing your mother's voice or cuddling with your cat make you feel safe, do those things more often. Feeling safe helps us relax. If you can, avoid situations where you feel you are in danger.

• Spend Ten Minutes Every Morning and Every Night Doing Deep Breathing Exercises

 Inhale for a count of four, exhale for a count of four. Or, put one hand on your chest, one on your belly, and deep breath through your nose. Try alternate nostril breathing, where you hold the right thumb over your right nostril and inhale deeply. At the peak of inhalation, close off the left nostril and exhale through the right nostril. You can also try a long, slow inhale, and then a quick, powerful exhale from the lower belly.

• Write Poetry

Write a poem, read uplifting poetry or choose an author and read all their poetry, either to yourself, aloud or start a poetry reading group. Some great poets include Walt Whitman, Maya Angelou, Robert Frost, Langston Hughes, Elizabeth Barrett Browning, William Shakespeare, Robert Browning, Henry Wadsworth Longfellow.

• Get Your Hands Dirty

That's right—research has shown that touching dirt relieves stress. Plant some flowers, grow a potted herb garden, dig up some weeds, plant vegetables, flowers, grass. Just put your hands in the dirt and enjoy.

• Spend More Time in Nature

Many studies have been done on the healing effects of green space on reducing stress and tension. The natural world offers some of the best relaxers available. Levels of serotonin, a neurotransmitter that regulates our moods, rise when we are outside in nature. Make it a goal to be outside at least 15 to 30 minutes a day, even if it just means sitting on the front steps of your apartment or in your driveway.

Smell nature, stare at nature, sit in nature, and be in the moment with nature.

Go barefoot. When you are unable to get outdoors, take some pictures of natural scenes and display them in your home or workplace, so you can enjoy the peaceful serene feeling being in nature can bring.

Take daily walks in a park. Sit under a tree. Put your hands in the dirt and garden. Sit on your front lawn and take in the sunshine. Bring a sketchpad to a park and draw. Feed the birds, the deers, the seagulls, the turkeys. Hike a local trail every morning. Choose a spot and stare at a tree. Sit on the beach. Lay down in the grass. Have a picnic at a local lake. Swing on some swings. Read a book outside. Grow some grass in a pot and sniff it. Touch a tree. Pick up some pine needles, or sticks.

• Bring Flowers Into Your Life

Buy yourself flowers weekly. Various studies have shown that we feel less negative and more energized when we are around flowers. At some local supermarkets, bouquets of flowers can often be enjoyed for $5 or less.

Put flowers in a visible place where you can see and enjoy them, such as by your bed, on the kitchen table, or on your desk at work.

• Hum Your Way to a Baby

Music can be a powerful tool in lifting our moods and relaxing our bodies. Music has been used as a healing tool for thousands of years, and it can be a healing therapy for you too. Research has shown that music sets off a neurological chain in the body that alleviates stress and induces relaxation.

As you undergo infertility treatments, begin using music as a way to relieve stress and elicit feelings of joy and hope. Commit to bringing more music into your life. Buy and play music from happy times in your life. Play music that lifts you up or relaxes you.

Avoid sad, depressing music that makes you melancholy or reminds you of sad events in your life. Play Broadway show tunes, inspirational music, music that you love to dance to.

Play whatever type of music calms you and helps you feel happy. Try some classical music. Play Italian love songs at dinner.

Keep a stereo in your living room or kitchen, and listen to music while cooking dinner.

Replace half an hour of TV watching each day with a half an hour of listening to music. Write a song or lyrics to a song. Play music when you feel worried or anxious, start listening to music as a way to distract you. If you play an instrument, sit down and play along to a favorite artist or song. Create a favorite play list you can listen to while driving to the infertility clinic.

If you've had formal music lessons, take out your instrument and play for your own enjoyment. Or purchase a set of drums, a piano, an organ, a flute, keyboard, or a guitar and just bang away. Let yourself enjoy creating sound for nothing more than the joy of creating sound.

Take some time to find the music that makes you feel like nothing can stop you. Play music that makes you feel like you are on a winning momentum. Research various forms of classical music to see what best suits you. If there is a certain instrument that you love, make sure to get music highlighting that instrument's sound.

Join a drumming group, take piano or clarinet lessons, sign up for a music course at a local college. Get a CD with the sounds of the ocean, wind or other forms of nature. Listen to musical theatre if it puts you in a great mood or study the works of a favorite band, singer of composer.

• Watch What You Watch

If the evening news brings you down, stop watching it for now. Horrible images, frightening scenes, upsetting events, are not going to help your body heal and become strong. If you get news updates on your phone, stop them if they shake you up and leave you depressed.
There is some evidence that when you are sad, your adrenals become weakened, which impacts the entire hormone system in your body.

From now on, watch movies and TV shows that make you laugh and generally leave you with an optimistic, positive, upbeat feeling.

When you feel happy, you have a better chance of keeping your adrenals strong. Organs, such as the thyroid can also be weakened by a sad mood. If not keeping up with the news makes you feel guilty, realize that you are just doing it during this time in your life. It is important to give your body a chance to feel safe and watching unsettling events that attack your feelings of safety is not what your body needs right now.

• Begin a Mild Exercise Routine

Find an gentle exercise that gets your body movingl. Nothing too demanding or harsh. Walk three or four times a week for a half hour.

Note here: once you do an IVF cycle, I would suggest stopping all extreme swimming, running and aerobic work-outs. This is not the time to push your body too hard with aerobic, running, or cardio-work-outs. Extreme exercise at this time will not aid your body in conceiving, but could negatively impact the outcome of your infertility treatments.

• Reduce the Time You Spend Looking at Screens

Too much time on your phone, computer, television, video games affects melatonin production and throws off the circadian rhythms that lead to deep, restorative sleep. As much as you can, reduce the time you spend with the technology in your life. Don't text as much, watch as many movies or TV, or play as many video games. Try to cut your screen time down in half.

• Move the Stress out of your Body

Take walks, dance in your living room, get a massage from a trauma release specialist.

For more information on reducing stress, Dancing Your Way to Fertility can be purchased at Amazon.com.

Chapter 11: Freeing Your Body from the Traumas and Painful Memories That Might Be Destroying Your Fertility

Our body is a walking history of our life. There is always a very strong and direct relationship between your emotional life and your physical health. You may not realize it, but trauma and painful experiences in your life can impact your fertility in a very significant way.

Your body contains and records all the traumatic and painful experiences you have endured. It then stores these traumas and sad memories in your cells and tissues.

Traumas, from rape or incest, to being bullied, criticized or rejected, can form negative pockets of energy in our cells and organs. Our bodies remember and trap feelings of fear, sadness, rejection, loneliness, betrayal, abuse, or disrespect in our cells. Our vitality and overall health is severely weakened once these negative pockets of energy inhabit our body.

Even if a trauma occurred long ago, its negative energy can remain stuck in our cells for decades.

Our brain produces neuropeptides in response to our emotions, and these peptides interact with the cells in our body, firmly connecting our mind, emotions and body. The feelings and thoughts then trigger physiological responses in our body that affect the chemical and neurological balance of the hormones involved in reproduction.

Never underestimate the brutal and destructive power that traumatic and upsetting life experiences can have on your fertility.

Since everything we have experienced since birth accumulates within us, to regain our health and fertility, we need to release and let go of these trauma pockets in our body that weaken us.

By releasing trauma pockets in the body, we are giving our body a chance to be restored to its true fertility potential.

When you release trauma, you are giving your body a chance to let go of the negative energy pockets stuck in the body.

Once these negative energy pockets are released, our bodies are free and unburdened from energy-draining emotions like hurt, anger, grief or shock.

Letting go, moving forward, forgiving ourselves and others, are all part of the release that is needed so that the traumas stuck in our body can no longer impact our infertility in a negative way.

Do not ignore this aspect of healing. You might have gone through a trauma or an extreme emotion that is altering the state of your body and ultimately stealing your fertility.

Here are some ways to rid your body of the traumas, painful memories and destructive emotions that could be interfering with your body reaching its maximum health potential and your right to have a baby:

• One of the best and most powerful ways to release and unblock emotional traumas that have physically lodged themselves within your cells and tissues is through body work. Various forms of holistic treatments are available that can unblock emotional traumas. These include: chiropractic adjustments, myofascial release, cranio sacral therapy, Somato Emotional Release, deep tissue massage, trauma release massage, neuromuscular therapy, Neuro Emotional Technique, Thought Field Therapy. Zero Balancing, therapeutic touch, reflexology, kinesiology, fascia release, trauma touch therapy, Somatic Experiencing, EFT, therapeutic body work, emotional release bodywork, or light therapy. You can do an online search using these terms, adding your city or town, to see what is available in your area.

• Consider applied kinesiology, a very powerful form of trauma release. It can be done by a kinesiologist, chiropractor or other holistic practitioner skilled in kinesiology, also known as applied kinesiology.

First, write a list of the traumatic and painful events you have experienced in your life, including names of the people who have hurt you. Give this list to a kinesiologist and ask that they muscle test each item on your list. If the kinesiologist finds that you are storing trauma associated with a certain person or experience, they can then apply an activator instrument that looks like a small, hand-held gun type mechanism, to release the emotion or trauma at its location in your body. This is a non-invasive treatment that can help you let go of long-held traumas and painful memories. If you have gone through a lot in your life, you may want to consider doing at least three or four treatments, or going on a weekly basis.

• Homeopathy and flower essences can be used also as a way to release traumas within the body.

• Write the experiences and events in your life that caused you a great deal of grief, trauma and fear, put them in an envelope, seal them and say goodbye to them. Mail them to an unknown address or to yourself. In these letters, say what you need to say and stand up for your right to voice out loud whatever you feel needs to be said.

Your memories do not have to stay locked up inside of you. You have a right to write letters stating the truth of your pain. Even if you blame yourself or think whatever happened is your fault, trust me, whatever happened is not your fault—and feelings of shame need to be sent on their way—because you have a right to your emotions, a right to your anger, and shame no right to keep you prisoner any longer.

• Write down all your painful memories, burn them in a fire and bury the ashes. You can do this outdoors in a fire pit, a bonfire, or in an indoor fireplace. You can do this alone, or with family and friends. Whatever you choose, it is a chance for you to physically see the end of the painful memories in your life. As they burn, consider these memories as disappearing so now you can allow health, happiness and vibrant fertility in your life.Throw the ashes of these memories into the ocean, a lake, or bury them. The hold these traumas have over you is now gone.

• Write a letter to yourself that gives you permission to say goodbye to your painful memories. When writing this letter, show love, compassion, forgiveness, and kindness to yourself. Let yourself know it is safe and okay to let go of the traumas of the past—that you are not safe by holding on and reliving these traumas over and over again. Let yourself know that you are not to blame for these events, nor should you keep holding yourself hostage to their power because of misguided shame you might be carrying.

• Pray about these old memories and ask God that their hold on you be released so that your body can heal and move forward.

• When you swim, walk or work-out, imagine that you are releasing and sweating away toxic, negative patterns in your body.

For example, if you are taking a walk, with each step repeat: I am walking away from my pain, I am walking away from my pain, I am walking away from my pain. If you swim, with each lap affirm: My traumas are floating away. My traumas are floating away. My traumas are floating away.

Or you could say: My hurt is being washed away, my hurt is being washed away, my hurt is being washed away. Exercise can be a way to physically release emotional pain.

• Write letters to the people in your past who hurt you or let you down. You never have to mail them, but in writing to them, you will energetically be releasing some of your pent-up feelings. Pour out your emotions, especially if there are people or incidents you think of often. Don't do this exercise if you have already moved past painful incidents in your life, because regurgitating old memories sometimes resurrects the pain and makes it worse. But if you find anger, sadness or other emotions pertaining to these incidents coming up often, then it is time for some cleansing and releasing. Don't be embarrassed that you are still hurt by an incident that occurred decades ago, or one that may not seem significant to others. If it hurt you and you still think or dream about it, then it deserves to be acknowledged and released.

We humans feel deeply, and we should not be ashamed of our sensitivity, our emotions or the impact that negative, toxic people and events can have on our lives.

• Volunteer to help others who have suffered or been violated in the same way you were. Helping others is a very powerful way to heal yourself. For example, if you are a victim of some form of childhood abuse, find a way to help other victims of abuse. Or if you need to heal from bullying, volunteer to help stop bullying in your area. Empowering and helping others is a form of taking back your own power. By using your energy and insight to heal others, you will also begin to heal yourself.

• Write a play starring yourself as a main character and tell the story of how this character releases her sad memories and goes on to give birth to a beautiful baby.

You may want to act out this play before very trusted family and friends, or it might be a play for you alone to enjoy. Either way is fine. Just remember: don't be afraid to write a happy ending to this story.

• Buy a bouquet of balloons, write your painful memories, tape them to the balloons, and then let them go one-by-one, saying goodbye to the negative impact these events had on your life.

• Plant a garden and name each flower a positive emotion growing within your body, such as joy, self-love, self-acceptance, an ability to see beauty, or an ability to experience joy. As your flowers grow, see them as a physical manifestation of the positive emotions growing within you.

• Write a song about the memories that weigh you down, but be sure to end the song with your letting go and moving past these memories, and on to the life you desire, surrounded by your children.

• Get a pet and talk with your pet daily about the memories that hold you prisoner. Keep an image that your pet is listening, silently healing you and unconditionally accepting you.

• Pray, pray, pray. Then pray some more.

• Have a conversation with yourself, making sure you know that whatever trauma you went through is not your fault. I repeat: NOT YOUR FAULT. Write a letter to yourself making sure that every part of you knows IT IS NOT YOUR FAULT.

• Write to characters in literature or history and tell them your life story. Select characters that you feel may have experienced some of the same difficult experiences you have. Ask for their advice and support in moving on to the next stage of your life. Then, write back to yourself as these characters, giving you support and advice

• Take a dance class and utilize the motion of dance to release toxic emotions.

• Paint a picture of the emotional pain that lives inside your body. Name the pain.

As you paint, let your inner knowing come forward to paint where your cells have stored these traumas. Use colors that express your pain. Paint pictures of the energy trapped in your cells being healed. Paint positive images of peace and joy entering your cells and tissues, allowing your fertility to blossom within you.

• Aim to forgive. Aim to forget. Aim to accept all the imperfections in this world and still see the beauty around you. Aim to forgive even those who don't deserve your forgiveness. You might start a forgiveness journal, and each day write: I forgive _____, I forgive _____. Allow yourself to feel the relief and joy that forgiving another—even someone totally undeserving—can bring. It is understandably hard, but you deserve a future free of the pain and anger that not forgiving will bear upon you.

• Buy or make yourself a blanket of safety. Make a blanket that symbolizes being safe—using colors, pictures, images, quotes and fabrics that give you a feeling of safety. You could make a blanket with pictures of people and places that soothe you and make you feel loved. Use material that you find pleasing and welcoming to touch. Or buy a blanket that appeals to you—it can be a kid's blanket, a lovely floral blanket, a big cozy blanket—and call it your 'safety' blanket. Sew some words on the blanket, such as 'It Is Safe For Me To Have A Baby' or 'I am Safe.'

For more on freeing your body from the traumas and painful life experiences that might be destroying your fertility, Dancing Your Way to Fertility can be purchased at Amazon.com.

Chapter 12: Letting Go Of the Secret Thoughts and Hidden Beliefs That Might be Holding You Back from Getting Pregnant

You may find this hard to believe, but hidden within your subconscious could be some negative perceptions of pregnancy, childbirth and motherhood that are holding you back from having a baby, without you even knowing it.

You may have some hidden fears or beliefs about becoming a mother that conflict with your desire to have a baby.

Sometimes, the body can hold two very different desires at once. One part of us wants one thing, another part of us wants another. Consciously, you may want to become a mother more than anything in the world. Subconsciously, you may have fears that are making it hard for your conscious wishes to come true. These two very different parts of you could be playing a tug of war: who will win? Who will get their way? Whose needs will be met? This conflict can make it hard for us to really commit and do the work needed to get what we want. This tug of war steals energy away from what your body really needs to be doing—and that is healing and getting pregnant.

Ultimately, the goal should be that all the different parts of you are working harmoniously together and have the same goal: to conceive a baby.

Deep fears and childhood issues sometimes need to be acknowledged, listened to and healed so you can move forward in having a child. It is important that you discover and acknowledge all your feelings and beliefs about becoming a mother—even the ones that are not all warm and fuzzy. Our conscious self might want something, but if our subconscious does not want it, it could be off doing a dance of its own. If your subconscious doesn't want something, your body could follow suit.

Subconscious fears about pregnancy, child birth or raising a child could even at times influence your hormones and the physical processes required for conception.

Does having doubt, fear, or hesitance about having children mean you won't be a great mother? Not at all. Millions of great Moms once had doubts or fears about becoming a mother. Millions more worried about pregnancy, childbirth and how their life would change. Embarking on a new life path naturally brings up feelings of doubt and fear.

To find out what your subconscious really thinks about getting having a child, start by asking yourself what you think about becoming a mother, and then write down whatever response comes from you without editing yourself. Allow your subconscious to voice its feelings on the subject without judgment or criticism.

Negative feelings or beliefs left unexpressed or unresolved hold considerable energy which can block conception. If you ignore your subconscious, it might stage a rebellion within your body—not allowing you to get pregnant because it wasn't given the respect and attention it deserved.

Begin by writing: "I will become pregnant soon" or "My womb is ready to receive" and then after you write that, start writing whatever comes up from deep within. Let whatever comes up from within you come up, come out and be heard. Write without editing or judging what you are writing. Do not consciously think about what is coming up, or try to force something you don't really feel or think. Just write.

This exercise can help you uncover what you are feeling about your infertility on many levels. It can also reveal if there is a part of you that wants to sabotage your efforts to become pregnant, or feels that you are not worthy of a baby. By knowing your innermost feelings, you can then work on bringing together the different emotions within you, so that you can achieve your goal. Later on, reread what you wrote and thank your subconscious for opening up.

Try not to judge your subconscious, even if what comes up is not exactly what you want to hear.

You could also write down the words: 'I deserve to have a baby' and then type or handwrite whatever comes up. Remember: No judging. No editing. No thinking this out. Write without restraint and let your deep internal self say what it needs to say.

Other writing prompts include:

• My body is ready to conceive and give birth to a baby
• It is safe to have a baby
• I deserve to have a baby
• I am good enough to be a mother and give birth to a baby
• My body is capable of giving birth
• A woman like me deserves to be a mother
• I am ready to be a mother and have children
• It is safe for me to become a mother
• Being a mother is a good thing for me

Honestly listening to every part of yourself shows your courage, because you are not going into denial.

Every part of you needs deserves to be listened to so they can all work together. If you ignore the needs of your subconscious, it could sabotage all the hard work you are doing to get pregnant.

Here are some questions to ask yourself, write responses to, and spend some time thinking about.

• **Are you afraid of repeating the same mistakes your parents made?:** Do you fear repeating some of the negative and dysfunctional family patterns you grew up with? Do you sometimes find yourself thinking, 'when I become a parent, I never want to do to my child what my parents did to me' or 'I never want to put my kids through what my parents put me through.'

• **Are you scared of becoming a mother?:** Do you have fears about becoming a mother, such as or 'I'm afraid of who I will become when I have a child' or 'I'm afraid I don't have what it takes to be a good Mom' or 'I'm afraid I won't be able to care for my child properly.'

• **Are you worried about losing some of your me-time once you have a baby?:** Are there aspects of your life that you really like that you are worried you will lose once you have a baby?

• **Do you fear that once you become a mother, you will turn into your own mother?:** Did your Mom behave or act in a way that you don't want to repeat and hurt you a lot as a child? Or did your Mom do things that you promised yourself you would never do? Did you long ago make a silent pact with yourself that you would never become your mother?

• **Do you sometimes feel infertility is a deserved punishment, either from yourself or from God, for something you've done or didn't do, in the past?:** Could infertility be something you think you deserve to suffer? Did you do something, or not do something, you believe merits you being infertile?

• **Do you feel God is mad at you?:** Do you feel God is judging you harshly for something you did in your past that you still feel guilty about?

• **Were you a victim of physical, sexual abuse or emotional abuse? Did you have an abusive parent?:** Do you ever fear that you will become an abusive parent like they were? If so, you might fear repeating negative family patterns.

• **Did you ever experience a trauma that has left you feeling unsafe and weary of new experiences?:** Are you open to new experiences or does doing something for the first time unnerve you? Do you often feel scared and worried about your safety?

• **Are you a bit of a control freak?:** Do you need to control everything in your life? Or are you able to let life flow naturally towards you? Does the idea of having a baby make you feel too out of control? Are you the type of person who needs to control everything in your life, and letting life happen is not something you are comfortable with?

• **Do you feel you really deserve a baby?:** Or do you feel unworthy of this joy? Is there something about who you are, or what you have done or experienced in life, that makes you think someone like you doesn't deserve a baby? Do you feel worthy of getting what you want?

• **Does yearning for something feel more natural and comfortable than actually getting what you want?:** Have you spent a lot of your life yearning? Are you the type of person who feels more comfortable when you are yearning, wanting or suffering over something you can't have?

• **Are you more comfortable when you are the one giving, rather than the one receiving?:** Do things like getting a gift or a compliment make you feel uncomfortable? Are you in the habit of being able to be on the receiving end of things?

• **Do you feel confident in your body's ability to give birth, or did you ever suffer an illness or injury that has shaken your belief in what your body can do?:** Do you see your body as weak and incapable? Have you ever suffered from a trauma or an illness that has left you doubting your body's strength and capability? Does physical pain of any sort bring up bad memories for you?

• **When you think of being pregnant, does the word 'fat' come to your mind?:** Do you consider pregnant women beautiful or unattractive? Do you fear losing your shape or physical beauty once you have a baby? Do you fear that pregnancy will ruin your body? Do you see pregnancy as an empowering event for your body or something that will steal the hot body you are proud of.

• **Does the work of caring for a baby seem overwhelming? Are you afraid of the demands that a child will make on your life?:** Do you ever see mothers with their children and think 'I could never do all that work.'

• **When you hear the word 'mother' do positive or negative images come to your mind?:** Do you associate the title 'mother' with positive, loving images or negative, frightening images?

Do you think of the positive words associated with mothers, such as loving, protective, warm, or do you think of the negative connotations surrounding motherhood sometimes promoted in the media, such as being controlling or demanding?

• **Do you fear going through childbirth or did your mother go through a very hard delivery with you?:** Do images of a woman screaming in pain come to your mind when you think of childbirth? Did you grow up hearing horror stories about your own birth? Did your mother talk a lot about the difficulty she had giving birth to you or a sibling? Do you have any negative thoughts about childbirth, due to media images or experiences of family or friends?

• **Did your own mother enjoy having children or did she complain about how hard it was to be a mother?:** Did you grow up with a mother, or a father, who found being a parent very difficult? As a child, could you sometimes sense how frustrated or overwhelmed your parents were with raising children? Did their experience taint your view of parenthood?

 • **Do you fear that your body can't survive childbirth? Does being pregnant or giving birth seem dangerous to you in any way?:** On some level, do you fear you might die during childbirth? Do you think being pregnant hurts? Do you have concerns about the physical dangers of child birth? Do you see woman as being in danger when they are pregnant or give birth?

For more on letting go of the secret thoughts and hidden beliefs that might be holding you back from getting pregnant, Dancing Your Way to Fertility can be purchased at Amazon.com.

Chapter 13: 50 Creative Projects To Help You Tap Into Your Fertility

Creativity is a powerful anecdote to feelings of hopelessness and depression. Doing creative activities can help you unlock and release negative energy patterns and paths in the body. Tapping into your creativity can help you transcend emotional blockages that may exist within your body.

Exploring your creativity can relax you, de-stress you, and give your body a dose of happy, healthy chemicals that can assist in healing infertility.

Here are some creative exercises and activities to try while undergoing infertility treatments:

1. Make a collage representing birth, babies, and the body's ability to conceive and have a baby.

You'll need a poster board, construction paper, or whatever kind of paper feels right to you. Cut out pictures from magazines, books, newspapers, or download and print pictures from the Internet of babies, pregnant women, along with images and words that represent what getting pregnant and having a baby means to you. Then, glue them in whatever pattern you choose on the paper or poster board of your choice.

When I was trying to get pregnant with my second child, I made a huge collage that affirmed my body's ability to get pregnant. I cut out pictures of babies and words like "the princess has arrived" and "mother love." I used lots of positive words that meant a lot to me and I personally connected to having children. My collage had pictures that represented new life emerging and the upcoming and most definite arrival of my child. I hung it in my office so I could look at it and feed off its positive energy every day.

Making this collage was a very joyful experience for me, because I had been trying for over a year to get pregnant and was not successful.

I was extremely depressed, but while making the collage, I entered a very optimistic and hopeful state of mind. Every time I looked at my collage, I felt renewed hope and a surge of power—something that I needed desperately to gain back at that time. A few months later, I did become pregnant and gave birth to my beautiful son.

So, collage away. I used a huge poster board which I felt made my collage something powerful to look at. Make sure to use whatever images, pictures, words strike a personal note for you.

2. **Make a collage celebrating babies.** Cut out photos of babies from magazines and write something at the top like: Welcoming All Babies— Including Mine! Or: Welcome To All The Babies and My Baby Too! Put a picture of yourself in the middle of this collage along with something that represents your baby's arrival. In doing this, you'll be setting out the welcome mat for your baby's arrival and reminding yourself that babies are born everyday and soon yours will be too!

3. **Make a collage on the topic of fertility.** Use words and pictures that represent your body enjoying a healthy state of fertility. If you see pictures that symbolizes fertility to you, add it to your collage. Make sure to put a picture of yourself in the middle of the collage, with words like: "My Body is Fertile" or "The World Around Me Is Fertile and I Am Fertile Too" or "I Am Part of A Fertile World." Surround your picture with powerful and meaningful images of fertility that you can personally relate to.

4. **Create a scrapbook titled "My Successful Journey To Motherhood"** and include in it whatever pictures, quotes, experiences or items reflect your story of having children.

5. **Go to a crafts store and purchase pink and blue buckets and make flower arrangements that you will have in your hospital room when you have a baby.** Get flowers and decorations that you want in your room when you have a baby.

6. Play inspiring music, like the theme to the movie 'Rocky', and march around your living room, picturing your ovaries turning out a healthy baby. Play music that puts you in a state of positive expectation and joy. Allow the music to help you transcend all doubt, if even for just a few minutes. Let the music carry you into a state of being where you allow yourself to feel your dream of being a mother coming true. Play a song that represents triumph and victory as you see yourself giving birth and becoming a mother. Then, as you play this song, move, march, dance in a celebratory way that says: my baby is on the way to me soon.

7. **Make a collage of all the goals and dreams in your life that came true, as a hefty reminder that good things do happen to you and will happen to you again.**

By reminding yourself that you can get what you want, you'll be triggering the thought of 'it happened once, it can happen again.' Along with words and images of goals and dreams that came true, include a picture of yourself next to a baby and write on the collage, "my dream of having a baby is my next dream about to come true." Hang it in a place where you can see it often.

8. **Write a song about your victory over infertility.** Songwriting is a way to express your feelings about having a baby in a hopeful and positive way. Write and sing a song about the triumphant way your body was able to conceive and give birth to a baby, as if it already happened. Write a song inviting your baby to find a home in your womb. Write a song to your future child about all the wonderful things you will do together. You don't have to be musically inclined to pen a song that speaks of hope and the happiness that awaits you.

 9. **Cut out words that describe the strength of your body and glue them onto a large piece of poster paper.** Put a picture of yourself in the center of these words, which can include words like: Fertile. Reproducing. Wise. Strong. Healthy. Ripe. Hang it somewhere where you can look at it often.

10. Imagine you are a coach and let your inner fertility coach give you tips on how to get pregnant. See getting pregnant as a game and listen to what your inner coach has to say about what you need to do to win this game. You can ask your inner coach to create a playbook, with what 'plays' or actions need to be taken for you to win at this fertility game. Draw a picture of your inner fertility coach and write down your inner coach's five best pieces of advice, and hang it somewhere you can see it often.

You know more than you think and this is one way to tap into that inner knowing.

11. Make or buy a kite and write your wish to have a baby, attach it to the kite, and send the kite out into the universe. Or attach to the kite a message inviting your future child to come to you and let it go into the world. Create as many kites as you wish and send them off with whatever message about having a baby you want to send out into the world.

12. Write a story about the day your child is born. Imagine the sights, the smells, the sounds, of this beautiful experience that awaits you. Write about the faces you will see, the emotions you will experience, the feeling of touching your child for the first time. As you write, let your body feel the story as if it were a reality, that already happened.
Go into detail: what hospital will you give birth in? What words will your partner, mother, and doctor say to you on the day your child is born? What will you wear to the hospital? How will you pack your suitcase? Write as if it already happened.

For all 50 creative projects to help you tap into your creative reproductive energy, Dancing Your Way to Fertility can be purchased at Amazon.com.

Chapter 14: Making Your Home Into A Fertility Nesting Center

Transporting yourself to an island paradise tomorrow may not be possible, but creating a world at home that is a nurturing incubator for you and your baby is possible.

Your home can be a helper in your fertility. It can be a nest where you feel safe enough to conceive, receive, give birth and care for your babies.

Sometimes, just a simple change can turn a home into a loving nest: painting a room a color you love, putting a sweet teddy bear or cozy quilt on your bed, hanging a photograph that calms or inspires you.

Envision yourself as a mother bird preparing a nest for her eggs she must keep safe and warm.

Feeling safe and in a nest will help you at this time, since the body finds it easier to procreate when it does not feel threatened or in a state of fight or flight.

Look around your house and ask yourself: Do I like it here? Do I feel safe here? Do I feel like I can safely keep and 'hatch my eggs here'?

Try to find ways to make your living space one in which you feel safe and comfortable. This could include: displaying a tea cup or doll collection, hanging photographs of people, places and memories that leave you feeling happy and warm inside.

Create a room that reminds you of things you loved as a child. How about a shelf in your kitchen with Raggedy Ann and Andy dolls? Or a 'Disney Dreams Come True' room with memorabilia from the various Disney princesses if that is something you love.

Walk around your home and try to find ways to increase the feelings of safety, joy and comfort.

Even if you don't live in an ideal setting or particularly like where you live, there are small things you can do to make your home feel more like a warm incubator for yourself and your baby.

Start by looking around home, and ask yourself: where do my eyes spend most of their time?

Notice where your eyes go each day—during breakfast, dinner, where you watch TV, and try to make your where your eyes spend their time more conducive to positive feelings.

Whatever areas of your home get your 'eye' time offer key opportunities for healing.

For example, if you often find yourself sitting in a certain room, looking at a certain wall, could you hang a positive saying or beautiful picture that inspires you or just make you feel happy? Example: When I was trying to get pregnant, I hung a picture of a little girl playing with a bunny in my bedroom. The picture made me feel soft and hopeful, even during very painful moments.

Ask yourself: what could I bring into my home that would bring pleasure to my eyes, ears and body each day? Think about items you could put in your home that would bring you a renewed sense of joy every time you look at them.

In whatever ways you can, make your home a place of healing, a nest where you can rest and rejuvenate as you prepare to conceive, an environment where you can access the positive emotions within you.

Here are some ways to turn your home into a comforting nest for you and your baby:

• Color

What colors make you sparkle? What colors give you a feeling of peace?

Don't worry about what colors are popular or 'in' right now—think about how different colors make you feel and put colors in your home that give you the type of feelings you are looking for.

When I was trying to get pregnant for the second time, I realized that the yellow paint color in my living room annoyed me. I never felt quite right in the room. So we went to the big hardware store and picked out a beautiful tahiti green paint color—wow what a difference that made! My spirits lifted every time I walked in that room. Granted, it was an unconventional color and not one that an interior decorator might have recommended, but at that time, it suited my soul perfectly. In fact, most people who came to my home liked the yellow color better, but it was draining me. I needed Tahiti Green's vibrance!

Two months later, I got pregnant. The color of my living room, of course, was not the 'cure' for my infertility—but I do credit it with lifting my spirits and helping me on some level, which is exactly the point: every little thing you can do to raise your spirits and reduce your stress matters.

If certain colors lift your spirits, bring those colors into your life. Look around: could you paint your bathroom a brilliant orange, the kitchen a soft pink, your living room a relaxing lavender. Think out of the box. Are you in the mood for bright, vibrant colors, like green or orange that bring about a friendly, happy feeling? Some color experts believe the color orange can help balance the adrenal glands, red provides energy and vitality to the ovaries, and violet is nurturing to the pituitary glands. Pay close attention to what colors you are drawn to and then bathe your home in these beautiful colors.

• Photographs

Photographs are a powerful way to relive positive, happy memories.

Instead of keeping your pictures locked away in boxes, or on your phone, print them out, buy a few frames and hang them throughout the house. Take photographs of places in nature that soothe you and people that you love. Display photographs that are reminders of life's beautiful and joyful moments.

• Make Sure Your Home Is Healthy

While paying attention to the aesthetics of your home, take some time to investigate whether or not your home is healthy. An unhealthy home can contribute to your infertility. Is there mold or mildew in your home? Have an air quality test done in your home. Do you need to invest in a air purifier or HEPA filter system if you live in a high pollution area? Some studies hve suggested that the air inside most house is 5 to 10 times worse than the air outdoors. Does your heating system need to be professionally cleaned? Do you have professional lawn care services that might be bringing lots of pesticides and chemicals into your life? Do you live in an older home that could still harbor lead paint, asbestos or arsenic? Do you have cabinets, paneling, plywood, particle board, carpets or furniture made with volatile organic compounds (VOCS)? Are the carpets in your home full of chemicals that emit VOCS? Do you have moth balls in your home that contain the chemical paradichlorobenzene? Is there lead in your plumbing fixtures?
Do you use air fresheners that contain ethylene-based glycol ethers and terpenes? Could you have radon in your home or a carbon monoxide leak coming from a furnace, generator, or appliances? Be aware of the chemicals that you bring into your home and start using natural cleaners that are non-toxic or even make your own homemade cleaning products. Filter your tap water, use a vacuum cleaner with a HEPA filter to get as much dust as possible, and change your furnace filter often.

• Bring Nature Indoors

Did you know that just touching a houseplant prompts a relaxing response in the brain? Create an indoor herb garden. Put plants all around your house. Buy yourself flowers every week.

Note: if you have pets, do not bring in plants that are toxic and could hurt or kill them. If you have pets, you may want to consider a small greenhouse that your animals do not have access to.

For more ways to make your home into a fertility nesting center, Dancing Your Way to Fertility can be purchased at Amazon.com.

Chapter 15: Journal Your Way To Pregnancy

Journal writing is powerful way to release trauma and heal from infertility. It is a way to express and let go of painful emotions, and give yourself the gift of hope when you need it most. In this chapter, we'll discuss different forms of journal writing that will help you express, release, get in touch with, and heal from your innermost feelings.

To get all the journals and journal exercises in Dancing Your Way to Fertility, including Journal Writing Through Your Subconscious, Your Daily Happiness Journal, the Life and Birth Affirmation Journal and My Child & I Journal, visit www.amazon.com.

Chapter 18: Fertility Affirmations

Words have power. Words can help heal the body. Words can provide your heart with hope. Saying, writing, singing, and reading affirmations everyday can lift your mood and help you physically manifest what you most want.

Go ahead, begin affirming out loud that yes, you are going to have a baby! Yes, your dream of becoming a mother is going to come true!

Doing affirmations will give you a chance to take conscious control of your thoughts. No longer will negative thoughts have free rein to take over and demoralize you. You deserve to hear affirmations that positively announce the arrival of your baby. Affirmations will help you combat the negativity, frustration and fear that often accompany infertility. They will give you a powerful way to tap into joyful, hopeful emotions that you deserve to feel as you walk down this exciting life path.

To get the affirmations and affirmation exercises, the entire version of Dancing Your Way to Fertility can be purchased at Amazon.com.

Chapter 19: Your Personal Fertility Vision Statement

A personal vision statement is something you can read, record and listen to each day. When you listen, visualize what is being said so it can sink deep into your subconscious. Be sure to fill in your name.

Here is your personal vision statement:

It is a bright, warm, sunny morning and you are feeling really good. You walk outside, take a deep breath of fresh air, raise your arms to the sky and say thank you, thank you, thank you for my baby.

That's right, YOUR NAME_____, having a baby is easy for you. Your body and mind are ready, willing and VERY able to have a baby.

You smile, because being vibrantly healthy and super fertile feels good.

Really good actually.

You know on a very deep level that having a baby is good and right for you. You deserve this baby. You are completely and totally worthy of having a baby. You are capable of conceiving a baby, carrying a baby for nine months and giving birth, in the healthiest, safest, most wonderful way possible.

That's right, you are worthy of having children.

Because you ate so many healthy green vegetables, let go of the toxins in your body, and said goodbye to all the trauma, anger and sadness in your cells, you are now able to give birth to a baby whenever you choose.

That's right: you can have a baby whenever you want to. Today, next week, next month, whenever you choose. Your body has the power to conceive and give birth to a baby whenever you want it to.

To get the entire version of Your Personal Fertility Vision Statement, visit Amazon.com to purchase a copy of Dancing Your Way to Fertility.

Chapter 20: Letters To Yourself

During your fertility journey, there are times you will need to be your own best friend. Here are some letters that you can mail to yourself, or leave around the house when you need a lift or just a reminder of how strong you are. Be sure to begin each letter by filling in your name and then signing it at the end.

_____

Dear_____

Congratulations! You are on your way to getting pregnant! Every day, you are one step closer to being pregnant! Every day, your body is getting stronger. I see you getting stronger! I can feel how ready your body is to conceive a baby. You are ready to have a baby! That's right-- your body can easily have a baby now! Congratulations!

Love,

_____

Dear _____

I know with all my heart that you will give birth to a baby soon. Your dear sweet ovaries, dear healthy healthy ovaries, can produce ripe, rich healthy eggs. Actually, right now they are making healthy fertile eggs! Your ovaries know how to produce good eggs. They are right now producing eggs that will lovingly grow into your baby. Thank you ovaries! Thank you for giving me healthy eggs!

Love,

Dear_____:

You are ready to be a mother. I can see it—you are ready. Nothing in your past can hold you back from having a child. You deserve this! You are worthy of this! There is nothing to fear when it comes to becoming a mother. You can do this. Millions of women from various backgrounds, life experiences and families do this. So can you. You do not need to be perfect to be a good mother. Go ahead, let yourself have this. You deserve a baby.

Love,

_____

Dear _____

Your vagina, your dear beautiful healthy vagina, is ready to receive. Yes, sweet vagina, you are ready to receive. Thank you for welcoming my baby. Thank you for opening up and allowing my baby in. Thank you for being a safe place for my baby. I love you vagina. I love everything about you. Thank you for receiving my child and giving it a safe home to grow.

Love,

_____

To get all the Letters to Yourself in Dancing Your Way to Fertility, visit Amazon.com.

A Moment In Song

Something wildly odd and beautiful happened this afternoon in the parking lot at the supermarket. I was there to meet a friend for coffee, and arrived a little early. Stuck with about an hour to kill, I decided to just listen to the radio.

I started praying about having a baby, as I usually do whenever I have a spare moment.

While I was doing that, Will Smith's "Just The Two of Us" came on the radio. The song is a father singing to his son. The Dad gives his son advice about not swearing, remembering to say your prayers, and holding the door open for girls. I love this song, as you can feel the power of this father's love for his child.

As I listened to the song, a wave of joy came over me--like someday I would actually be able to sing this song to my child.

I imagined that on my child's wedding day, I would play this for him or her, and recount this moment in the parking lot where I was begging for his/her birth.

It wouldn't matter if my child was a boy or a girl--this song would still apply. "Just the Two of Us"--me and my child. I got so deeply into this vision, of me dancing and singing this song to my child at their wedding, that it began to feel completely real. Of course I will have a baby someday! No doubt..it will come to pass...

The song moved me to another time and place, and it felt so completely real, that it was as if it had already happened.

By the end of the song, I was on a wild high, visions of my child dancing in my head: their wedding, their birth, this song being our song. For a few minutes, I landed in such a place of hope.

A good place...

For those few minutes, all the desperation I usually feel was swept away by a tidal wave of faith and hope.

Do I dare think this song was maybe a kind of answer to my prayer?

For a few minutes even after the song ended, a feeling of certainty that I would have a child was mine, all mine.

My prayer, coupled with that song, brought me to a place of joy I haven't felt in a long time.

My child was real--our relationship was real--the future with my child in it all became real.

Could this be a signal?

I can't imagine the fullness I will someday feel if there was a little person on this earth I could actually sing and dedicate this song to.

For more diary entries, visit Amazon.com to purchase Dancing Your Way to Fertility and The Infertility Diaries.

Chapter 21: The Emotion of Deserving

Emotionally, it is important to root out every single thought that you may possibly hold about not deserving a baby.

If you are a person who s feels undeserving of good things, you might on some level not feel you are worthy of receiving a baby.

Many people say they want something, but on some level, they don't really think they deserve it.

Because of this deep subconscious belief, they prevent themselves from actually attaining what they want because a part of them simply doesn't think they deserve to get it.

For more on the emotion of deserving, visit Amazon.com to purchase the entire copy of Dancing Your Way to Fertility.

Chapter 22: Start Living Authentically

An often overlooked part of healing from infertility is living your life through your authentic original self.

Having a baby is a very natural, authentic process, and if you have buttoned up yourself to the point that doing anything real and authentic is absent, you may need to tap back in and welcome your true self.

You need to reunite with your true self so that you can feel completely at home in your body.

Feeling comfortable in your own skin and feeling at home in your body will help release inner reserves of energy, nourishment and peace that could help heal your infertility.

You have the right to embrace and welcome your original authentic self—even if you have ignored her for a very long time.

The authentic self is the 'you' at core of who you really are, not the 'you' people have told you that you are suppose to be.

Due to feeling shamed, judged or rejected, many women live their life through fake, imposter personalities because their true self was never valued or accepted.

The original self is buried—this beautiful, wise, helpful part of ourselves—is left dormant and ignored.

She deserves better. You deserve better.

Starting today, listen to your real self. Let her speak. Pay attention to what she wants and needs.

For more on living authentically, Dancing Your Way to Fertility can be purchased at Amazon.com.

Chapter 23: Welcoming Your Mother Within

Within you lies a mother waiting for the moment when she can step forward and assume her rightly role. In many ways, you are probably already stepping forward into the role of a mother by the way you live your life. You have most likely done many things that demonstrate the maternal part of you. It is likely that you already have had the experience of mothering yourself and those around you. So Mom, let it show—you know you are already living and breathing this role that is rightfully yours.

Here are some ways to get in touch with your inner mother:

• Begin today to see yourself as a mother. When you look in the mirror, remind yourself that yes, you are a mother, and it is only a matter of time before your children physically manifest themselves. Say aloud: I am a Mom. Picture being called 'Mom' or write: I am a Mom.

• See yourself surrounded by children. They are smiling. They like you. They like to be with you. Visualize yourself surrounded by children often. Picture yourself enjoying your children, talking with them, playing, and doing things you know come naturally to you. When you picture yourself with your children, visualize it authentically—if you hate to bake, don't try to conjure up an image of yourself baking. Maybe you would rather be racing your children down the beach instead, or teaching them to use a hammer or repairing a fence together. Maybe you love to read, and reading to your children is something you will cherish. Or maybe you want to put on some roller blades and coast down some trails with them. There are a million different ways a million different mothers enjoy their children.

• Write down all the qualities you already have that you associate with being a mother. Examples can include: being responsible, kind, tender, generous, strong, ingenius, creative, courageous, honest, a hard worker, loving, understanding, gentle, funny, fun-loving, responsible, resourceful, directed, nurturing, a leader, active, empathetic, self-sacrificing, playful, self-disciplined, fun.

For more ways to welcome your mother within, the entire version of Dancing Your Way to Fertility can be purchased on Amazon.com.

Chapter 24: Hitting Bottom

There are moments in infertility that are so painful, that trying to give advice about how to cope with them almost seems disrespectful.

So I will apologize right now for even attempting to give advice on how to get through moments so devastating that there is really no solace.

The pain of not conceiving is not something to be taken lightly, or something that some best-ten-tips list can cure.

I have suffered that kind of pain. Pain so raw and disappointing, and so completely upsetting to life's balance, that any advice given on how to deal with it can feel trite and disrespectful.

Infertility can attack the core of a woman's intrinsic and basic sense of what is natural and right. When having a baby does not occur naturally, it can rock to the core the way a woman feels about her life in general.

For a woman who desires children, not being able to reproduce can sting like a bloody violation of one of the most basic human rights.

So in your most painful moments, remember this: if you desire to be a mother more than anything, you will find a way to be a parent, either biologically or through adoption. Your misery will fuel you to do whatever you need to do to become a parent. Your intense pain may be the reason you agree to undergo yet another IVF, and it may be that one more try that wins you the baby of your dreams.

Or that misery may push you to adopt an adorable baby and still try for a biological child.

All I know is no one wants to stay in the stalemate of misery indefinitely, and if you can't stand this feeling, then be glad for a moment, because that horrible feeling will push you to do things, try things, continue things, open yourself up to things, and never give up on things that could very well bring the child of your dreams into your life...as long as you don't give up and get stuck in the misery.

Please understand that anyone so desperately sad about not having a child is desperately needed in this world. You are needed in this world.

A person who is a lover of children is a treasure. This world desperately needs people who want to parent and who love children, and will do anything for that privilege and responsibility. This world needs people who feel that children are a sacred trust, worth all the sacrifices, and not a burden.

And it isn't fair that you have to wait so long for that child you want.

Your attitude toward having children is very different from those who see children as annoying nuisances who do nothing but drop crumbs on the floor, rather than the sacred gift they are.

For that kind of pain, you deserve an applause, a standing ovation, a huge golden trophy, a million hugs.

I have lived through the wretchedness of feeling you are being robbed from the life and family experience you always imagined yourself having.

I have walked that road of bitterness, anger and frustration so intense that nothing I have ever experienced compared to the utter misery of not being able to conceive and bear a child.

Having a child is a right every woman is born with, and to not be able to fulfill this inherited natural human right is beyond painful and grueling. When I reached my lowest points of misery, I sobbed without shame on the steps of an old run down donut shop in an ailing, decrepit town.

On another occasion, after learning I was not pregnant, I cried so much that my neighbors overheard me and were convinced my husband was beating me.

Once, I was so distraught after an IVF that didn't work, I left 12 messages on the voice mail of my nursing team at the clinic asking question after question about what might have gone wrong.

So I'm assuming you will be a lot saner in your darkest moments than I was. But if you are not, that is okay and completely understandable too. You will find a way to survive this, thrive and fulfill your need to love and care for children. Just remember a few things:

• **Keep Believing:** Never stop believing that something good is about to happen. The ability to keep hope alive and keep a believing attitude even during the darkest moments can motivate you to keep trying.

Never stop seeing and visualizing that baby you long to hold. Picture it, envision it, talk to it, believe that little sweet human is coming. Hold on to hope even when it looks like you should give up. Act as if it already happened. Each morning, step outside your door, raise your hands to the sky and say, "I am ready to receive a baby" or "thank you. I am ready to receive my baby." When you wake up each morning, whisper, "I am pregnant." When you get out of bed, walk like you are pregnant, act like you are pregnant, and repeat the words, "I am pregnant. I am pregnant."

• **Use Your Anguish To Generate Change:** Nothing motivates a person to action like intense emotional pain. When the pain is so bad you can't stand it, you will also be hitting a powerful emotional point: Stay open. Answers can come when you are in this type of pain. You may be willing to go the extra mile that you were unwilling to go before.

Your pain can be the motor that keeps you going--so as bad as it feels, don't hate it. Great revolutions and profound historical changes have often been propelled by those in so much pain, they had no choice but to force change and make life better. Your pain will force change too.

You will find a way to fill that vacuum inside you--as long as you don't let the pain crush you, stop you, or submerge you into a helpless pit.

When you are in that kind of pain, you will be faced with two choices--either you can fall into a pit of despair and drown, or you can kick and scream and demand that something different happen.

Every day, make one choice that will move you forward and bring you one step closer to your dream. Choose action over inaction. That way you won't be permanently stuck in the pit of despair.

• **When You Have Reached What Seems Like A Dead End, Take An Unexpected Turn in the Road:** Go left. Go right. Start over and do it again. Close your eyes and walk backwards.

Try to think about getting pregnant in new ways, analyzing the situation from various perspectives. Picture yourself sitting at a table with the world's greatest minds: what advice would they give you about your infertility? Be open to the ideas that come. Pretend someone else is in your situation, and ask yourself: what would your inner, say, Oprah Winfrey, do in this instance? Or your inner Eleanor Roosevelt? What advice does your inner Einstein have for you? How about Dr. Phil or Ghandi?

• **Go To A Trauma Release Specialist:** Your body needs to release all the pain and trauma that can result from enduring infertility. Find a chiropractor, kinesiologist or myofascial release expert in your area who specializes in body work or trauma release. Write a list or a paragraph of what you have gone through and give it to the trauma release practitioner. Let them work on releasing whatever traumas are lodged in your body. By doing this, you will be freeing up some energy so you have the stamina it takes to continue infertility treatments.

• **Read Inspirational Books and Listen to Inspiring Music:** Put your mind's focus on what inspires and uplifts you. Bring hopeful music and books into your life. Fertilize your soul with positive words and happy outcomes.

• **Pain Can Destroy You or Motivate You to Win:** Don't let your pain immobilize or debilitate you. Instead, use your pain to propel you to action.

Let your pain be a motivator—not a destroyer. Use your pain to help you determine what is happening within your body. Then, let the pain of wanting a baby motivate you to make the changes necessary for your body to get stronger and better able to conceive a child.

• **Understand that Your Drive to Parent Will Find a Home in This World:** An empty space does not stay empty forever. Voids find a way to be filled. Your fervent desire to be a parent will seek until that desire is filled in some way. You will be a mother. You will make it so. That empty space inside you will be filled. You will find a way.

For more on how to cope with infertility when you feel like you are hitting bottom, an entire copy of Dancing Your Way to Fertility can be purchased at Amazon.com.

Part II: Secondary Infertility

Chapter 27: Coping With Shots and Injections

Enduring injections is part of the infertility process. The first time I did it, I worried about it all day. As the time came closer to the 'shot', I felt like I was trapped in some type of dreaded countdown. It never really became easy, I found ways that made it bearable and sometimes relatively painless.

Here are my best tips for coping with injections:

• **If your husband or someone else is giving you the injection, have something interesting that you can read sitting in front of you.** For me, I put a beautiful book on bed and breakfast inns in front of me. The lovely blue cover on the book soothed my soul. It was pretty and sweet, and represented everything that getting an injection wasn't. Looking at it was an escape: I'm not about to get a shot…I am visiting a lovely bed and breakfast inn and about to have homemade blueberry muffins, jam and a cup of tea. Right before my husband would insert the needle, I would turn to a recipe in this book and start reading it. Somehow, doing this helped me get through the many nights (and years) of shots.

• **Put on a favorite song, some comforting music, or a real party song.** Close your eyes and sing-along.

• **My opinion: Don't look.** Especially if the shots scare you, it is best not to look. Close your eyes and look away.

• **I am an expulsive person.** I like to talk and expulse my feelings. For me, it helped to exhale through my mouth a few breaths during the shot. Using my breathing as a release always helped me.

• **Open a candy bar or some favorite food and smell it, take a bite.** Distraction works. A delicious chocolate, a song, a book—get your senses engaged in something else during the injection.

• **Remind yourself that the discomfort you might experience is going to be worth it.** Give yourself something to look forward to when it is over.

Chapter 28: How To Protect A Cherished Pregnancy

If you have had recurrent miscarriages, you might want to:

• Ask to have an infection screen of your vagina.

• Ask for a Vitamin D deficiency test.

• Ask for a mineral deficiency test.

• Get tested for antiphospholipid syndrome (APS) which causes blood clots to form. A doctor can treat this condition with a low dose of baby aspirin or injections of heparin, which is a blood thinner.

• Visit your dentist and make sure there are no infections in your teeth or gums.

• Let your doctor know if you have any chronic conditions, such as thyroid disease, epilepsy, lupus, or a family history of clotting disorders.

Ways To Protect Your Baby and Prevent A Miscarriage Once You Are Pregnant

First off, it needs to be said: sometimes you can prevent a miscarriage and sometimes you can't. Most of the time, you can't. If you do miscarry, please know it is not your fault. Nature does this more often than we realize. Even in past generations, many women suffered miscarriages, they knew nothing about. There are some things you can do to protect your growing baby, but please be aware that it is not your fault in any way if a pregnancy does not continue. The pain, of course, is immeasurable and intense, and there are no words to gloss over the immense sense of injustice and sadness this awful loss brings. Please, if possible, do not give up in trying again if you have endured this great loss.

Here are some things you can do to help maintain a healthy pregnancy:

• Boost Your Progesterone Levels

Maintaining adequate progesterone levels is absolutely key when you are pregnant. Ask your doctor if progesterone is something you should take to reduce the risk of miscarriage. If you have miscarried before, you might want to request progesterone from your doctor. Progesterone plays a role in maintaining the uterine lining, and because of this, some researchers have theorized that low progesterone plays a role in causing miscarriage.

Taking Vitamins C and B, and minerals such as zinc and magnesium, can help the body produce progesterone.

Foods that help raise progesterone levels include: walnuts, bananas, wild yams, spinach and kale. Pumpkin, watermelon, chickpeas and squash seeds, which are high in zinc.

Try to avoid getting yourself in a stressful 'fight of flight' situation, which tends to reduce progesterone levels.

Avoid all foods and herbs that can increase levels of estrogen, such as dong quai, hops, lavender, licorice, tea tree oil, and red clover blossom.

• Keep Your Thyroid Healthy

If you have had recurrent miscarriages, you may want to have your thyroid tested to be sure you are maintaining a TSH above 2.0. Foods that encourage a healthy thyroid include artichokes and pineapple, which offer natural sources of iodine. Other foods to help the thyroid include garlic, sunflower seeds and turkey, which are high in selenium, and flaxseed, that contain high levels of Omega 3. Copper and iron rich foods are also very important to thyroid function. These include cashews, leafy greens,and lean red meats. Avoid Bromide, a chemical found in fluoride and chlorine, that disrupts the endocrine system. Bromide can also be found in soft drinks, plastics and some hair dyes. Also avoid soy, which some health practitioners believe can weaken the thyroid.

• Nurture Your Kidneys

In Chinese medicine, it is believed that if a woman has suffered a miscarriage, she needs to work on her strengthening her kidney Qi. Start by drinking lots of water. Try to avoid situations that bring up feelings of fear. Eating deep red foods like red bell peppers, red grapes, cranberries and beets, that can help rebuild and replenish the kidneys. Blueberries and apples are also good for the kidney. Avoid fluoride, artificial sweeteners and fructose. Avoid root canals and exposure to toxic mold, along with pesticides and toxic cleaning products.

• Be Aware Of Your Homocysteine Levels

High levels of homocysteine can be a threat to your growing baby. Homocysteine is a sulfar-containing amino acid that can cause your blood to clot more easily. Be sure your prenatal vitamin has adequate levels of B6, B12, and folic acid, because this combination of B vitamins has been shown to prevent miscarriages that are caused by high homocysteine levels.

• Avoid Excessively Stressful and Sad Situations

As much as possible, try not put yourself in situations that bring up extreme and intense feelings of fear, stress or sadness.. Stress tremendously affects the hormonal stability within the body. Let yourself sleep more, relax and say no to increased responsibilities and work at this time.

Avoid people, situations and activities that bring up a strong 'fight or flight' response. Limit time spent in situations where you feel nervous, anxious and uncomfortable. Do not listen to sad music or watch movies that bring up feelings of grief. Deep breath and give yourself permission to relax.

Never underestimate how powerfully grief, sadness and toxic connections with others can impact your hormones.

• Keep Your Hormones Stable

Keep your blood sugar levels stable, eat lots of leafy greens, don't exhaust your adrenal glands through stress or lack of rest. Foods that help balance hormones include olive oil and berries. Avoid white flour products, sugar, caffeine and alcohol.

• Make Spinach Your Best Friend

Eat lots of spinach, it offers a rich form of iron that is needed for healthy **cellular division.**

• Find Out If You Have Celiac Disease or Are Gluten Intolerant

Gluten, found in rye, wheat or barley, has been known to cause miscarriage in those who are allergic.

• Take Your Minerals

One study linked a history of miscarriage to low levels of magnesium. Symptoms of magnesium deficiency can include agitation and anxiety, restless leg syndrome, sleep disorders, irritability, nausea, vomiting, abnormal heart rhythms, low blood pressure, confusion, muscle spasm and weakness, hyperventilation, insomnia, and even seizures. Foods high in magnesium include spinach, brown rice and pumpkin seeds.

• Make Sure You Are Getting Enough Iron

Lack of iron has been reported to cause miscarriages. You may want to talk with your your doctor or nutritionist about taking an iron supplement. Food sources of iron include red meat, turkey, chicken, kidney beans and chick peas. Be sure you are taking Vitamin C to help iron absorption.

• Take Baby Aspirin

Some studies have shown that taking one baby aspirin a day can reduce the risk of miscarriage. Ask your doctor about this. One of the benefits of baby aspirin is that it prevents blood clots that can cut off nutrients to the baby and prevents preeclampsia.

• Be Alert To High Or Low Blood Pressure

Be sure you are aware of your blood pressure levels. Avoid fried or processed foods, deep breath and get plenty of rest. Repeat the word 'relax' several times a day.

• Keep Blood Sugar Levels Stabile

Avoid sugar and do not let your blood sugar levels fluctuate. Your goal while pregnant is to maintain stable blood sugar levels. Avoid white flour, carbohydrates and sugar products that spike blood sugar levels.

• Consider Taking Coenzyme Q10 Supplement

Research has shown that women with low levels of coenzyme q10 are at an increased risk of miscarriage.

For more on How To Protect A Cherished Pregnancy, the entire version of Dancing Your Way To Fertility can be purchased at Amazon.com.

And A Fibroid Would Have Been So Easy.....

A ton of bricks. Falling on me. Right now.

I went for my first check-up since the fibroid operation.

My doctor very calmly and with no apology whatsoever, told me I did not have a fibroid after all.

Oops.

That explains my amazing recovery. It also explains why I could walk so well after supposedly having a large fibroid removed. It explains why all the pain I was told I was suppose to feel after the operation never came.

And here I was thinking I was some kind of medical marvel.

I'm very confused right now.

The doctor didn't seem upset by her findings.

Or embarrassed.

Or even slightly apologetic.

She told me as if it was no big deal. So I reacted like it was no big deal, because I didn't want to make her feel bad for making such a stupid mistake.

If no fibroid existed, then why am I having so many problems getting pregnant a second time? Now I have no easy answers. The fibroid gave me a way to understand everything.

I am back to square one.

Does this mean I went through all that worry, nausea, and postponement of my IVF for absolutely nothing?

I had thought that changing doctors was a good idea, especially when she discovered a baby-eating fibroid. I thought, 'finally, someone has found the root of all my infertility problems."

As it turns out, she diagnosed me incorrectly.

Now I have to wait until September to do another IVF. Every month that passes means my eggs are one month older.

Having a fibroid made it all so black-and-white.

When I told friends I had a fibroid, many reacted with 'oh yes' 'ah ha' and 'that explains it' and I was told story after story of their sisters, best friends, and co-workers, who had trouble getting pregnant, discovered they had a fibroid, had it removed, and soon had babies born without a hitch. There wasn't something deeply wrong with me on some unexplainable cellular level! It was all the fibroid's fault.

Simple.

Nope. As usual, nothing is that simple.
I have no fibroid. No easy explanation to hang on to. An apology, or an oops, I led you down the wrong path these past few months, would have been nice.

When I thought a fibroid was at the root of all my problems, I sometimes felt slightly carefree. I thought my infertility problems were now going to be simple and straightforward: I have a fibroid. It is killing my babies. It needs to be taken out. Once it is gone, all will be well.

Now I'm left to think that maybe our daughter was a one-in-a-million chance that won't happen again. I feel an almost overwhelming grief.

I want to think this doctor knows what she is doing. She was named by a magazine in our area as one of the best infertility doctors in New England. I like her personality and I trust her.

I just hate that because of this operation my IVF was postponed. I also hate that I had to go through all that pain. For what? For nothing? I told everyone I had a fibroid, even the alternative practitioners I was working with, which might have impacted the treatments they chose to use on me.

And a fibroid would have been so easy...

For more diary entries, visit Amazon.com to purchase Dancing Your Way to Fertility and The Infertility Diaries.

Chapter 30: How to Maximize Your Chances For Conception The Days Before and After An IVF

Before

• Consider additional acupuncture treatments close to the time you are doing an IVF. Ideally, increase the number of acupuncture treatments the week of the IVF to two to four. If you can, have one also done the day before the procedure. Perhaps if you go once a week, consider increasing your appointments to two to three times within the seven days before an IVF. Research has shown that acupuncture improves blood flow to the ovaries and uterus, relaxes uterine spasms, and relaxes the nervous system.

• In the weeks prior to an IVF, make sure you are eating well. This is not the time to splurge on foods with lots of sugar, trans fats, msg, or white flour. Consider increasing the amount of vegetables you take in, such as spinach and garlic.

• Green tea is linked to increased fertility. The polyphenols and hypoxanthine in green tea can increase the percentages of viable embroyos. Some studies suggest drinking treen tea can also help eggs become more fertile.

• Increase the amounts of healthy fat you consume. In a recent study, women who ate avocados, a healthy monounsatured fat, were more likely to conceive a child after IVF. Other healthy fats include olive oil. Avoid saturated fats and trans fats as much as you can, ideally entirely, for two to four weeks before IVF.

• Be aware of the help certain supplements can provide, such as coenzyme Q10, which in some studies have shown to improve egg quality. Some studies have shown that women taking coenzyme Q10 had higher fertilization rates in IVF than women who weren't taking the supplement. Some studies also show that coenzyme Q10 deficiency can sometimes cause miscarriage.

• Increase your time spent in the sunshine to 30 minutes a day if you possibly can. Even if it is cold out, try to be in the sun more than usual amount of time. Perhaps bundle up and sit outside. Sunlight increases levels of Vitamin D, which is key to balancing sex hormones in women and improving sperm count in men, according to various researchers. In cold northern countries, the rate of conception increases during the summer months, according to some studies. If you are doing an IVF in the summer and you live near a beach, park or lake, consider spending more than the usual time outside in the sun.

For more information on how to maximize your chances for conception before and after an IVF, visit Amazon.com to purchase the entire version of Dancing Your Way to Fertility.

Diary Excerpt: Sunday Retrieval

Today was the egg retrieval.

We got to the hospital about 6 a.m. A kindly nurse at the desk welcomes us. For a moment, the whole place feels different—a fantasy island of fertility where surgical procedures are pink and beautiful. For a few minutes, I am lulled into actually believing this might turn out to be fun.

We were the ones on the floor that morning and we are put in a room at the end of the hallway. It is so quiet. I am not deceived by the wallpaper anymore. Now, it all feels very serious and very real, just like it did the other two times. I pray and pray. I always feel a measure of fear when I'm going under anesthesia. And heaviness. I feel a heaviness when it comes time to do an IVF, as if the weight of the world is on me.

Finally a young man comes to wheel me down to the OR. I have seen him before. He has wheeled me to several operations and procedures. He doesn't remember me, but I remember him. He must see a thousand like me each month.

In the waiting area, I am put me in front of station 3.
Three? Could it mean..a sign that I am going to have triplets!!!!!

I let myself get a bit giddy imaging that this IVF will result in triplets. Triplets....Imagine! The instant large family of my dreams! My little girl suddenly blessed with three siblings! Three sisters? Oh my God, four girls!!!! Or maybe two girls and a boy? Oh my God, a family of three girls and one boy! Two boys and a girl? Then I would have two girls and two boys! Four children would be a lot of work at first, but my kids would never be lonely. I am imagining our family photo twenty years from now. All four kids and then someday all their kids will have babies and their kids will have lots and lots of cousins. In my old age, I'll always have a child to be with. I'll be busy with kids until I'm 58 years old!

I let this fantasy play out in my head and I am feeling happier and happier.

Triplets!

A few minutes later, I am wheeled into the operating room. The anesthesioligist is kind, and very quickly, I am asleep.

I wake up, I don't know how much later, in that horribly awlful waiting recovery area. But good news—I am told retrieved ten eggs! Ten! Oh my God! Ten!

All my hard work trying to get healthy paid off. I can't believe this. I probably will end up with six good eggs, and then there is a good chance that three of those six will take, and I will have triplets!

Can you imagine? My daughter will never be lonely. She will always have at least one sibling in the house to play with.

In three days, my eggs will be implanted back in me. Ten! I'm betting triplets are on the way!

Day of Transfer

Today was the transfer of the embryos, where they implant the eggs mixed with my husband's sperm back into me.

I ended up with three eggs, not ten, but three.

Dr. M, the one who so devastated me a few months ago by saying my eggs were bottom of the barrel, was ironically, the doctor on hand for the procedure. As always during procedures, she was kind, generous and nurturing. I've figured out that she is good at handling tests, but not to have as the primary doctor on your case. Maybe she likes the non-pressure of just stepping in for a procedure, without the pressure of having to follow-up and figure out what is going on.

Dr. M. said it was wonderful that I did everything the clinic asked of me, submitted to all the tests they recommended, including a balloon test known as a hysterosalpingogram that was not too pleasant. I just smiled, pretending to be laid back about the whole thing.

She never could have guessed how much she devastated me a few months ago.

She seemed to have no anger or resentment over the fact that I dumped her and switched to another doctor. Maybe she is so busy, she didn't even notice that I had switched doctors at all. Or she was just relieved to be rid of a patient who was creating too much work for her.

Anyways, as she was just about to do the transfer, she said it was bad luck to have the same doctor do a transfer twice, especially since the last transfer she did didn't work out. So she went to get another doctor to insert my eggs. I was grateful for her sensitivity, especially since she was the one whose words made me feel so hopeless.

Before she went to get the other doctor, she took an ultrasound picture of my eggs and said, "Let's hope this is a first baby picture." Hopeful and kind words, and made me feel good. Imagine if this was my baby's first picture. She smiled kindly at me, and for a minute, I think I can forgive her for the pain she caused me.

The other doctor came in, did the transfer, and now I must wait and hope my baby comes soon.

Praying and Waiting

It is 5 o'clock in the morning. A light snow decorates the earth outside my window, and there are three embryos inside me fighting to live.

After changing doctors, eating according to blood type, taking two shots a day of some pretty powerful infertility drugs, going to acupuncture once a week, a myofascial release expert and a kinesiologist twice a month, I ended up with three fair-to-poor quality embryos.

If I have one baby, I will be glad. No, ecstatic. Overjoyed. Full of bliss and gratitude. Yet, there is a part of me who wants three babies, an instantly large family by today's standards. I am trying not to be stressed. I am trying not to think negatively. I am trying not to hate myself, but right now, self-hate is roaring through my body.

It seems no one in my life realizes how absolutely helpless you can feel when you've done everything medically possible both in conventional medicine and in alternative medicine and still end up with only three embryos.

Earlier this week, I made a collage representing pregnancy.

I got a giant poster-size paper and cut and glued pictures of babies and mothers and words like 'revel in your ripeness' 'miracle' 'prayers' and 'mom knows cool.' My collage is beautiful and I hung it in my office.

I love this collage. I look at it and think: 'it is possible. I could make a baby.'

For now, however, I'm going to cheer my little embryos on.

"Dear Embryos,

I don't know you yet. One of you, or all of you, may end up being one of the most important persons in my life. You may end up being the answer to my prayers. I may someday get to hold you and love you.

You may grow and become more than I ever imagined. Right now, know I love you. I love you if you make it and I love you if you don't make it. I am cheering for you. I am trying to give you the best parts of me. I am your mother and you are my children, and I'm hoping we can take that connection into the physical realm. Take what you need to take from my body. Feed off me. Ignore my tired, cranky spirit. Ignore the self-hatred looming inside of me. Ignore all the mixed emotions that are stirring around in my head. Just hear this: you are loved. You are wanted. You will be given as much as I can give. Your sister Amber needs you. Your Daddy Chris is praying for your continued growth. I, your mother, sit nervously and tenuously, hoping Dec. 20 comes quickly and the answer is yes. Please, please, please, let the answer be yes."

www.ingramcontent.com/pod-product-compliance
Lightning Source LLC
Chambersburg PA
CBHW081350280526
45788CB00009B/2830